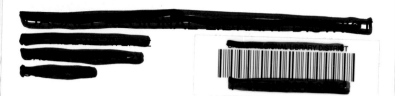
DATE DUE

NY 29 '02		
AG 31 '02		
MAY 1 5 2003		
JE 03 03		
GAYLORD		PRINTED IN U.S.A.

Other books by Robert S. Ivker, D.O.

Sinus Survival
Asthma Survival
Arthritis Survival
The Self-Care Guide to Holistic Medicine
Thriving

Headache Survival

THE HOLISTIC MEDICAL TREATMENT PROGRAM FOR MIGRAINE, TENSION, AND CLUSTER HEADACHES

Robert S. Ivker, D.O.
with Todd Nelson, N.D.

Jeremy P. Tarcher/Putnam
a member of Penguin Putnam Inc.
NEW YORK

Most Tarcher/Putnam books are available at special quantity discounts for bulk purchase for sales promotions, premiums, fund-raising, and educational needs. Special books or book excerpts also can be created to fit specific needs. For details, write Putnam Special Markets, 375 Hudson Street, New York, NY 10014.

Jeremy P. Tarcher/Putnam
a member of
Penguin Putnam Inc.
375 Hudson Street
New York, NY 10014
www.penguinputnam.com

Library of Congress Cataloging-in-Publication Data

Ivker, Robert S.
    Headache survival : the holistic medical treatment program for migraine, tension, and cluster headaches / Robert S. Ivker, with Todd Nelson.
        p.   cm.
    Includes bibliographical references and index.
    ISBN 1-58542-141-3
        1. Headache—Alternative treatment.   2. Holistic medicine.
    3. Headache—Prevention.   I. Nelson, Todd.   II. Title.

RC392 .I95   2002   2001054198
616.8'491—dc21

Printed in the United States of America
10   9   8   7   6   5   4   3   2   1

Illustrations by Maud Kernan

To the millions whose lives are governed by headache

ACKNOWLEDGMENTS

I'd like to thank my publishers Joel Fotinos and Phyllis Grann for offering me the opportunity to write the five-book Survival Guide series and choosing to include *Headache Survival*. Given the prevalence of headaches, I'm grateful for the chance to help many millions of headache sufferers while enlightening them about the remarkable health benefits of America's newest specialty—holistic medicine. My literary agent, Gail Ross; my editor, Mitch Horowitz, and his assistant, Allison Sobel; my coauthors of *The Self-Care Guide to Holistic Medicine,* Bob Anderson and Larry Trivieri; and my wife, Harriet, have all made significant contributions to this book.

The bulk of the information comprising the Headache Survival program was derived from the pioneering work of Ken Peters, a friend and holistic physician. Since 1995, he's been teaching me the holistic medical treatment for headaches that he's developed during his more than twenty years as an internist. My colleague, Todd Bezilla, did an excellent job of writing the bulk of the section on osteopathic medicine. And once again I am most grateful for the valuable contributions of Todd Nelson, a naturopathic physician who coauthored both *Arthritis Survival* and *Asthma Survival.* We've become quite an effective collaborative team, and working with him has made writing this and the other books an especially pleasurable process.

CONTENTS

HEADACHE SURVIVAL

INTRODUCTION
HEADACHE SURVIVAL

Only when we are sick of our sickness shall we cease to be sick.
—LAO-TSU, from the *Tao Te Ching*

Do you know anyone who has never experienced a bad head-ache? Not surprisingly, headache is among the most common chronic conditions afflicting Americans. This book will present the holistic medical treatment for the three most common types of chronic recurring headaches—*tension, migraine,* and *cluster.* Headache, regardless of what type, is usually a message your body is sending you that there is an imbalance in your life. Holistic medicine addresses each aspect of life—body, mind, and spirit—while utilizing both conventional and complementary therapies to prevent and treat disease. But most important, the focus of the practice of holistic medicine is on creating a state of optimal well-being. The goal of *Headache Survival* is for you to learn to use the symptom of head pain to experience physical, environmental, mental, emotional, spiritual, and social health. To create this condition of holistic health, the *causes* of chronic illness are treated just as aggressively as the physical *symptoms.* If you become an attentive observer of the triggers for your headache (and this book will assist you in this training), you will learn a great deal, not only about the causes of your headaches but about the nature of the imbalance in your life. You will become much more effective at treating as well as preventing your headaches. The primary therapeutic modality in mitigating the multiple factors responsible for causing headaches is *love.* The fundamental principle underlying America's newest specialty is: *unconditional love is life's most powerful healer.* This book will help guide you in a process of learning to love and nurture your body, mind, and spirit, while simultaneously offering you many options for quickly relieving and preventing headaches.

Although I have spent the majority of my time during the past fifteen years treating chronic sinusitis, allergies, and asthma, in recent years as migraine headache has become a more incapacitating and prevalent problem, I have devoted more attention to the treatment of this condition. That research has led me to consult primarily with Todd Nelson, N.D., a naturopathic physician with whom I've coauthored *Arthritis* and *Asthma Survival,* and Ken Peters, M.D. Both are significant contributors to the Headache Survival Program. Ken is a holistic internist and medical director of the Northern California Headache Clinic in Mountain View, California, and has focused on headache treatment for the past twenty-one years.

The prevalence and increasing severity of headaches reflect a societal problem in twenty-first-century America. We simply spend too much time in our heads! Our brains are far too overworked, just as we are, and *brain strain* is rampant in the United States. Although both migraine and tension headache are hereditary, it is not genetics that has caused headache to become such a common problem. Our lives are imbalanced, with nearly 40 percent of adults reporting that they work sixty hours or more a week. This group gets by on only six hours of sleep a night. In fact, a recent poll by the National Sleep Foundation found that the more time you spend at work, the less sleep you obtain. Almost two-thirds of our adult population gets less than the optimum eight hours of sleep. This data has a profound impact on understanding the most significant causes of the epidemic of headache in America. Most physicians agree that *stress is the primary cause.* But what is the specific nature of that stress? It probably has most to do with performance anxiety, which is often coupled with the intensity of our quest to achieve more and more. We're spending more hours working (the average work-week is now forty-six hours); a lot of that time is spent sitting in front of a computer (which emit unhealthy positive ions), while processing far more information than the average brain is meant to handle. We've heard for years from the neurophysiol-ogists that the average person uses only between 5 and 10 per-cent of their brain. They also estimate that we average 50,000 thoughts per day. That means if we sleep for seven hours, then while we're awake we're consciously thinking an astounding *one thought every second!* It is also estimated that 95 percent of those thoughts are the same ones we were thinking the day before. Our minds, and specifically only a small area of the brain, are working nonstop. Is it any wonder that our heads ache? We des-perately need to give our minds more rest, to redirect our think-ing into less stressful physical, recreational, and creative pursuits, and to rebalance our lives. This is the essence of the holistic approach to treating headaches and the Headache Survival Pro-gram.

Every chronic dis–ease represents a state of imbalance and dis-harmony. Whether it's headache, asthma, arthritis, or heart dis-ease, there is a restriction or obstruction in the flow of life-force energy through the body, mind, and spirit that stems in large part from *a deprivation of love.* Whether this lack of nurturing takes the form of poor dietary choices, breathing toxic air, not getting enough exercise, thinking negative or limiting thoughts, overworking at a job you're not enjoying, or not committing more time to your closest relationships, the basic problem is that you're not caring for yourself as well as you can. Holistic medi-cine is the most effective method I've found for healing any chronic condition, chiefly because it enlists the full participation of the patient in her/his own care. Applying and practicing each aspect of the Headache Survival Program will provide you with new opportunities for loving and nurturing yourself, which in turn will rekindle your inherent life-force energy and facilitate healing.

This book is based on the model of holistic medical treatment for chronic disease that I originally developed in the best-selling book *Sinus Survival*. Both of these books describe a holistic approach offering you a comprehensive guide to a variety of therapeutic options. In the following chapters, information will be presented to help you treat, prevent, and heal your headaches as well as to experience optimal well-being. This will include:

- symptoms and diagnosis
- conventional medical treatment
- risk factors and causes
- holistic medical treatment and prevention, with recommendations for body, mind, and spirit (including *diet, nutritional supplements, herbs,* and specific *physical, psychological,* and *bioenergetic therapies*)

The primary objective of this book is to teach you how to use your headaches to initiate a healing process that will guide you to a state of optimal well-being. Love, self-nurturing, and rejuvenation are the therapeutic tools you'll need to attain your goal. This condition is limiting your ability to think clearly and creatively, and is significantly diminishing your capacity to enjoy life. I'm assuming that's why you bought the book. But, in addition to reversing the symptoms of headache, it will be possible for you to experience a condition of *holistic health*—to feel better than you have in many years, while you relieve the recurring episodes of severe pain.

Bear in mind, as you begin to implement this holistic treatment program, that true healing is far greater than simply the absence of illness. The most effective way to cure any chronic illness is to *heal your life,* not just repair your physical dysfunction, which in your case is headache. Therefore, I strongly advise that you use most of the tools and information provided in Chapters 3, 4, 5, and 6—"Holistic Health: The Thriving Self-Test"; "Healing Your Body"; "Healing Your Mind"; and "Healing Your Spirit"—and not just simply rely on the Quick Fix presented in Chapter 1. What you learn in the latter chapters will assist you in strengthening your energy and vitality, and in increasing your awareness of the physical, environmental, mental, emotional, spiritual, and social factors that may be contributing to your headaches. The specific therapies provided in these chapters will then enable you to more permanently reverse the symptoms and prevent recurrences, rather than experience a temporary fix. *The holistic treatment of any chronic disease includes addressing and eliminating the multiple causes; adhering to a healthy diet; getting regular exercise; making affirmations, visualizations, emotional work, prayer, or meditation a part of your daily life; and creating intimate relationships.* As a result, you will become much more sensitive to what foods, thoughts, feelings, or people make you feel good, and those that make you feel more uncomfortable or even trigger your headaches. You can begin your training as a healer of headaches by initially following the recommendations in Chapter 1, "The Headache Quick Fix"; gaining a greater understanding of what each of the three most common types of headache are in Chapter 2; and taking the Thriving Self-Test in Chapter 3. Then you will be ready to start the Headache Survival Program in Chapter 4.

WORKING WITH YOUR PHYSICIAN

Although this book is intended as a self-care guide to healing headaches and creating optimal wellness, I recognize that many people will read it while under the care of a physician. I recommend that you use the suggested therapies as a *complement* to the medical treatment you may already be receiving, and urge you to inform your doctor that you are doing so. Nothing in this book contradicts conventional medical treatment, and *proper drug use under the guidance of your physician can be practiced safely in conjunction with the complementary therapies I provide, unless specifically stated.* Holistic physicians recognize that drugs and surgery play an important role in treating disease, and I have included a section on the conventional medical treatment for the three common types of headache. My therapeutic recommendations are based on the successful approaches that I, Todd Nelson, and

Ken Peters (cocreators of the Headache Survival Program), and many of our holistic medical colleagues use to treat headache in our clinical practices. They are not the only ones that work, but simply those with which we have had the most experience. By following these recommendations, over time you will experience considerable improvement with your headache condition, with great potential for freeing yourself of this oftentimes disabling affliction and feeling healthier than you ever have before. The comprehensive focus on healing all of the life issues that may be contributing to your headaches lies at the heart of the practice of holistic medicine and is the essence of the term *self-care.*

WORKING ON YOUR OWN

If you are not already under a physician's care, you might try starting with the holistic therapies on your own, unless otherwise indicated, and see how you feel after two months, before deciding to use conventional treatment or finding a holistic physician. And if you have been treated conventionally and conclude, after careful consideration and consultation with your physician, that the liabilities of the conventional treatment (such as dependency or unpleasant side effects from medication) outweigh their potential benefits, then commit solely to the holistic approach presented in the book, or take steps to find a holistic physician. One of the advantages of holistic medicine is that its combined use of complementary and conventional therapies often makes it possible to use lower dosages of medications to good effect, thereby minimizing harmful side effects.

HOLISTIC PHYSICIANS

If you are suffering from headaches (or any other chronic disease) or trying to improve the quality of your life, you may want the support of a holistic physician. You can find one in your area by contacting the American Holistic Medical Association (AHMA) on their website at www.holisticmedicine.org. to obtain their *Physician Referral Directory.* This list includes both physician members (M.D.s and D.O.s) and associate members (holistic practitioners other than M.D.s and D.O.s). The best resource for a referral to a *board-certified* holistic physician is the American Board of Holistic Medicine (ABHM). In December 2000, the ABHM administered the first certification examination in holistic medicine to nearly three hundred physicians, setting a new standard for quality health care in America. To locate a board-certified holistic physician (M.D.s and D.O.s) near your home, contact the ABHM at 425-741-2996.

PROFESSIONAL COMPLEMENTARY THERAPIES

The discipline of holistic medicine includes the prudent use of both conventional Western medicine and professional care alternatives, such as *ayurveda, acupuncture, behavioral medicine, Chinese medicine, chiropractic, energy medicine, environmental medicine, homeopathy, naturopathic medicine, nutritional medicine,* and *osteopathic medicine.* Chapters 4, 5, and 6 include mention of each of these therapies that have been scientifically verified as an appropriate professional care treatment for headache. To learn more about these therapies, see the Resources section, which lists the primary organizations that oversee each of these therapies and provides a listing of practitioners nationwide. Each of them is also described in the appendix of *The Self-Care Guide to Holistic Medicine,* which I coauthored with Robert A. Anderson, M.D. (the president of the ABHM), and Larry Trivieri, Jr. That book also presents the holistic medical treatment for sixty-five of America's most common ailments.

CHARTING YOUR PROGRESS

One way to monitor the progress of your holistic treatment program for headache is to evaluate your physical symptoms on a weekly basis. You can do so by using a chart similar to the **Symptom Chart** shown on page 56. This is an example of a headache symptom chart, and lists the most common symptoms you may experience if you suffer from migraine, tension, or cluster headaches. If you experience symptoms not included on this list, add them in the left-hand column and rank them from 1 (worst) to 10 (best or no symptom) on a weekly basis. You can also uncover possible emotional factors that are contributing to your condition by similarly ranking your emotional stress level each week. You should be able to graphically correlate higher stress with worsening physical symptoms. The same is often true with dietary factors. Also keep track, at the bottom of the chart, the medications, herbs, nutritional supplements, and other remedies you are using. **NOTE:** *The vitamins, herbs, and supplements recommended in Chapter 4 are available in most health food stores, and through Thriving Health Products. The suggested dosages are based on those that I, Ken Peters, and our holistic colleagues have used extensively in our clinical practices. These dosages may vary somewhat from the suggestions of your own personal holistic physician.*

By using the Symptom Chart you can more easily evaluate your progress and better determine what works for you and what doesn't. (Remember, each of us is a unique individual, with specific needs and requirements for maintaining health.) As you practice using this chart you'll become adept at the early recognition of dietary, environmental, and emotional factors that aggravate your headache, and be able to quickly respond with an effective therapy. The better you become at listening attentively to what your headaches are telling you about the imbalance in your body, mind, and spirit, the more effectively you will be able to *prevent* recurrences of your condition. This art, science, and discipline is the basis for the practice of both holistic and preventive medicine. As you continue your training and see the results, you will be less afraid of taking risks and making the needed changes in your life. You will develop into a highly skilled self-healer as you continually experience a greater degree of well-being. Although you may be starting out suffering with frequent and severe headaches, remember that the greater your *enjoyment* of this life-changing challenge, the better your results will be.

This book will enlighten and educate you: You'll learn why you've suffered for so long, and what you can do to improve that condition. But for the Headache Survival Program to make a profound difference in your life, you'll need to give yourself a gentle but firm push in the direction of optimal health—a condition of high energy and vitality, creativity, peace of mind, self-awareness, self-acceptance, passion, and intimacy. The critical ingredients for your success are a heightened *awareness* of your needs and desires (What do want your life to be like?); a *commitment* to providing them for yourself; the *time* required to incorporate new healthy habits into your life; and the *discipline* to stay on your course in spite of episodes of significant pain. These are the essential factors in learning to love and nurture yourself, and especially your strained brain. And it is also the primary objective of this holistic medical treatment program.

If you are willing to make the commitment, this program will enable you to *heal yourself of migraine, tension, or cluster headaches.* Although you might still have an occasional headache, they will occur less frequently, won't be as incapacitating nor last as long as they do now, or require your ongoing dependence on medication. More important, you will understand why the headache occurred, have the tools to treat it quickly, and avoid the debilitating and frightening experience of enduring such severe pain that you are unable to function for a prolonged period of time. But the most significant aspect of your healing process is that you will almost always learn or relearn a valuable lesson through your pain that helps to *prevent* subsequent headaches.

Although optimal health requires a commitment to a lifelong healing *process,* we live in an age of the quick fix. We've grown up believing that there's a fast and effortless solution to all of life's hardships. And if there is not such a miracle available today, it won't be long before science and technology provide it. But to heal your dysfunctional brain and blood vessels, while creating a balance of optimal well-being throughout every dimension of your life, requires a commitment to the Headache Survival Program comparable to one you would make if you'd just started a new job. *Healing yourself is the most important work you'll ever do, and the greatest gift you'll ever receive.*

After two months of making a commitment to this program, you will probably be "surviving" quite well, with a significant improvement in your symptoms. If you can maintain and strengthen that commitment to yourself, within six months you will be healthier than you've been in years, and within one year you'll be experiencing a state of well-being you've never known before. The most important advice I can give you is to take your time, be gentle and accepting of yourself, and know that there are no mistakes—only lessons. Study diligently, listen attentively, be willing to take risks, and have fun while you're at it. It's definitely a challenge, but the rewards are unimaginable!

—Rob Ivker
June 2001

THE HEADACHE QUICK FIX

After reading the Headache Survival Program in the introduction described as a *healing process* and not a *quick fix,* you may be wondering about the title of this chapter. I realize that upon embarking on a life-changing program requiring a strong personal commitment, most people in our society would like a simple and safe way to take the initial step. To facilitate change, you must first diminish the resistance that may arise from the anticipation of how much time you will need to invest in this program. If it is a high enough priority, you will be willing to take the time. You may also need to modify your attitude in approaching long-term dietary changes as well as taking dietary supplement pills on a regular basis. In addition, you might be confronting the fear of letting go of long-held beliefs and behaviors that have dictated the way you live your life. This insecurity is perfectly understandable. Therefore, rather than trying to do everything at once, which for many people can be overwhelming, this chapter will offer you several options for more *gradually* introducing this holistic approach into your life while experiencing relatively rapid **symptom improvement.**

The primary objective of the Headache Survival Program and the holistic treatment for any chronic disease is to heal the specific part of the body that is not functioning properly. The method for correcting this physical dysfunction is for you to nurture not only the diseased part but your entire body along with your mind and spirit.

This healing process usually begins on the physical level, because the body provides the most immediate feedback: telling you what feels good and what makes you feel worse. But if you're feeling some degree of headache all the time, it's not easy to determine what one intervention—an herb, dietary change, or relaxation technique—is doing for you. It has usually taken many months or years to produce the conditions creating your ongoing problem with headaches. Therefore it will take some time for your body to function well enough on a consistent basis and for you to begin to trust the signals and feedback it is giving you. By improving physically at the outset, you'll become much more aware of what you can do to heighten this feeling of well-being and what behaviors—what you're eating, how much you're sleeping, what you're doing that's causing you stress—make you feel worse. Over time you will learn to become your own best healer and develop reference points for what techniques work best for you. To speed the process of correcting the imbalances in your life, Todd Nelson, Ken Peters, and I have developed the initial **Physical** and **Environmental Health** Components of the Headache Survival Program, which are summarized in this first chapter. It won't be effortless, but if you're committed to healing and curing your headaches, this is the most effective way to begin your new full-time job. This approach will enable you to feel better as quickly as possible. Chapters 2 through 6 will help you to understand *why* all of these recommendations are included and better appreciate how they are helping to maintain and enhance your health.

We've found that if you stay on the complete regimen described in this chapter for at least four to eight weeks, you will usually be able to at least partially restore physical balance and experience considerable and often dramatic improvement. You should also be able to decrease the use of analgesics and any other medication you're presently taking. These physical and environmental health recommendations are explained in more depth in Chapter 4. The improvement in your physical condition should provide you the motivation to commit to and fully benefit from the Mind and Spirit Components of the Program while addressing all of the causes of your illness.

The practice of holistic medicine is based on loving yourself physically, environmentally, mentally, emotionally, spiritually, and socially. There is no quick fix in this lifetime process of experiencing optimal health. Since each of us is a unique individual, our prescription for *healing is based on self-awareness* and in understanding the specific messages your body is sending with each episode of pain. However, you can give yourself a jump start by closely following the majority of these initial recommendations, which work quite well for almost anyone.

In the following guidelines for treatment of specific ailments, you have the option of doing and taking everything right from the beginning or at any time of your choosing, and simply following the instructions in the table. The only risk that I'm aware of in starting out with the entire Program is that it could feel a bit overwhelming and may be more challenging to *maintain* the new daily practices than if you gradually ease into it.

Each of the different therapeutic options presented in the following outlines will contribute some benefit. There is no single remedy or magic potion that will quickly cure headaches. However, most people who are interested in this Program have been uncomfortable for many months, if not years. For them, taking two to four months to feel better than they have in a long time can be described as a *quick fix*.

After about two months of incorporating most of the physical and environmental health recommendations into your daily routine, you can begin the mental and emotional health components of the Program, followed in another one to two months by spiritual and social health. These facets of the Program will be described in Chapters 5 and 6. With each component you will be uncovering factors that have contributed to causing your headaches. Remember, the more often you experience a sense of physical well-being, the more acutely aware you'll become of what makes you feel good and what triggers the episodes of pain. This information initially will allow you to make healthier choices regarding what and how you're breathing and what you eat and drink. Your diet will make a significant difference, but as you progress you'll find that what you eat may be less important than what's eating you! You'll soon realize that the latter four aspects of health—comprising the *mind* and *spirit* sections—require far less of your time but a deeper commitment and greater awareness than the recommendations for the *body*. However, the more you can work on these less tangible but potentially more immune-suppressing and -enhancing factors, the more you will be able to effectively *prevent* severe attacks of headache, *reduce* or eliminate your analgesics and medications, and possibly *cure* yourself of chronic headaches.

Before you begin implementing the Physical and Environmental Health Component, please take the Thriving Self-Test in Chapter 3. Your Thriving score will help you to see where your life is unbalanced and what aspects of the Headache Survival Program will require the bulk of your attention. I would also suggest reading Chapter 4, "Healing Your Body," to gain a better understanding of why the therapies in the following lists are used. Many of the products included in these lists that are not readily available at most health food stores can be obtained by referring to the Product Index at the end of the book.

I'm assuming that the majority of you have been diagnosed by a physician and are aware of the specific type of headache with which you're suffering. If this is not the case, then refer to Chapter 2 and review the primary symptoms of each of the three common types and adhere to the following *quick fix* recommendations.

MIGRAINE HEADACHE

1. Keep a headache **diary** to determine your headache triggers (refer to pages 60 and 61).

2. **Diet**
   a. Avoid foods on the Headache Relief Diet (pages 96 and 97).
   b. Eat regularly and try not to skip meals.
   c. Drink a strong cup of coffee at the onset of symptoms—works best if you have not been consuming coffee as a habit.
   d. Stay well hydrated with bottled or filtered water.
   e. Take Pill Curing, patent Chinese medicine found in health food stores, for acute nausea. (Also goes by Gastrogen from the professional brand Metagenics. Available through your holistic physician.)
   f. Ginger tea could be useful for acute nausea.

3. **Environmental factors**
   a. Avoid rapid ascent to high altitudes.
   b. Avoid sunlight glare—wear U.V. protective sunglasses.
   c. Avoid air pollution, carbon monoxide, smoke and perfume scents.
   d. Sit in front of a negative-ion generator, and breathe deeply.
   e. Get absolute dark and absolute quiet/stillness!

4. **Exercise**
   a. Do aerobic exercise for approximately 30 minutes at least 4 days a week.
   b. Practice gradual warm-ups and cool-downs.
   c. Avoid dehydration—drink plenty of fluids.
   d. Avoid overexertion and overheating.

5. **Vitamin B$_2$** (riboflavin)—400 mg per day in the morning. (This dose can be taken for three to four months. Then reduce to 100 mg for maintenance.)

6. **Magnesium** (glycinate)—400 to 500 mg per day. (Up to 2,000 mg on day of onset of pain.)
   IV Magnesium @1,000 mg administered by your holistic physician can immediately relieve a migraine.

7. **Feverfew**—100 mg of standardized 0.7% parthenolide per day. Needs to be taken daily for maximum effectiveness.

8. **Petadolex:** Standardized Butterbur extract 2 pills per day—1 in the morning, 1 at night. Start immediately for long-term prevention, and to reduce frequency and intensity of headaches.

9. **Omega-3 fatty acids**—EPA (eicosapentaenoic acid) in a dosage of up to 300 mg 3✕/day for 12 weeks, then reduce to 2✕/day. In addition, take flaxseed oil, 1 tablespoon 2✕/day with meals, or 3 capsules 3✕/day with meals.

10. Get regular adequate **sleep**—avoid under- and oversleeping.

11. **Acupressure**—Apply pressure for 1 minute to the hoku, B2, and GB20 points (see figures on page 132).

12. **Aromatherapy**—Breathe from a facial steamer after adding a couple of drops of pure peppermint oil. The scent of green apples might also relieve pain.

Some women experience migraines at a particular time of the month. The most common are premenstrual and can typically be treated with a natural progesterone, magnesium (400 to 500 mg per day), and vitamin B-6 (150 mg per day). There are also mid-cycle migraines that correspond with ovulation and could be due to either low estrogen or an estrogen/progesterone ratio discrepancy. In this case, sophisticated hormone testing is recommended.

TENSION HEADACHE

1. **Environmental factors**
   a. Make sure your workplace is ergonomically sound and practice good posture. Avoid repetitive motion stress and strain, take frequent work breaks to stretch, and breathe. Avoid static postural positions, or being sedentary for long periods of time.
   b. Avoid long periods of time in front of a computer screen, and always keep a negative-ion generator running next to you to correct the ion imbalance (excess of

positive ions from the computer screen) and for clean air. Remember to have the ion generator pointed in the direction of the computer screen—from behind or beside you.

   c. Good ventilation and adequate oxygen.

   d. Belly breathing exercises to relieve tension and calm stress.

   e. Practice an anger-release technique regularly.

2. **Exercise**

   a. Do aerobic exercise at least 5 days per week for 20 to 30 minutes.

   b. Practice shoulder and neck exercises daily.

3. Apply **heat** or **ice** locally over areas of head pain.

4. **Aromatherapy**—peppermint oil, eucalyptus oil, and/or alcohol applied to the temples and forehead, 5 to 10 drops 2 or 3 times a day; or inhale from facial steamer.

5. **Herbal Muscle Relief** or **Herbal Muscle Relief P.M.** (an antispasmodic herbal preparation)—dosage can range from 2 tabs morning and night for prevention to 2 tabs every three hours for relief. The product contains magnesium, calcium, and the herbs: valerian, passionflower in Herbal Muscle Relief, and valerian, passionflower, kava, and hops in the Herbal Muscle Relief P.M. The P.M is designed to help sleep. (Available through Thriving Health Products.)

6. **Inflavanoid IC**—take 2 pills morning and night preventively, and 2 pills every 2 hours during acute headache. (This is an excellent combination of anti-inflammatory herbs that can take the place of NSAIDS. It is COX-2 inhibiting, reduces pro-inflammatory prostaglandins, and increases anti-inflammatory prostaglandins. A Metagenics product.)

7. **Neuromuscular therapy**—hands-on bodywork targeting relief of trigger point activity in trapezius, scalenes, SCM, etc., which may be causing referred pain to the head. Can be **self-applied:** Find tender points in muscles

of neck and shoulders, press into the point firmly for 8–10 seconds, then ease pressure and massage area in circular fashion. This helps break neurological pain reflex arc.

8. Medical evaluation for **adrenal fatigue.**

9. **Topical herbal analgesic**—apply herbal balm containing capsaicin, menthol, and other pain-relieving herbs; massage into neck after trigger points are treated.

10. **Kava kava**—if there is a history of anxiety, use this herb daily; Standardized to 30% kavalactones, 75 mg per tablet, take 1 tab 3× daily. (Metagenics Kava Plus is best—it combines kava with well-known Chinese anxiety-relieving herbs.)

11. **St. Johnswort**—if there is history of mild depression, use high-potency standardized @ .3% hypericins, 1 tablet 2–3× daily between meals. (Metagenics St. Johnswort Plus is best, as it has other anxiety-relieving herbs.)

12. **Deep relaxation techniques:** Meditation/visualization/imagery/progressive relaxation of muscle tension.

CLUSTER HEADACHE

1. **Diet**
   a. Avoid alcohol during the cluster headache cycle.
   b. Avoid nitrites such as aged cheeses, aged meats, chocolate, and MSG during the cluster cycle.

2. Apply **ice** or **heat** to the area of pain—whichever feels better.

3. Try a **hot shower massager** with moderate pressure on the scalp.

4. **Avoid** letdown stress, bright lights, and excessive cold or heat.

5. Try 100% **oxygen** at 7 liters per minute by face mask for 15–20 minutes while sitting.

6. **Magnesium** glycinate—400 to 500 mg daily or more. Also IV magnesium can be used under medical supervision.

7. **Melatonin**—6 to 10 mg nightly, only on medical supervision; may improve daily cluster headaches within 4 to 5 days.

8. **Hepataplex**—a traditional Chinese herbal compound; 2 pills between or before meals 3× daily.

Chapter 2

WHAT ARE MIGRAINE, TENSION, AND CLUSTER HEADACHES? WHAT CAUSES THEM? HOW DOES CONVENTIONAL MEDICINE TREAT THEM?

It is estimated that 45 million Americans suffer from disabling headaches that interfere with their lives. Headache accounts for over 80 million doctor office visits per year, and is the seventh-highest-ranked reason for seeking medical help. Nearly $500 million is spent on medications to treat this problem, while headache has become the second-leading cause of loss of worker productivity. The three most common types of chronic headaches are *tension, migraine,* and *cluster.*

Tension headaches are by far the most common type of headache (approximately 90 percent of all people seeking medical help for headaches), and perhaps the most common human affliction. Men and women are equally affected, as are all age groups. The pain is mild to moderate and is not debilitating. These headaches can last from thirty minutes to seven days but typically last from one to six hours. The quality of the pain is usually a dull, steady ache that feels like a band or a vise around your head. It is usually bilateral (located on both sides of the head). There is often associated tightness of the neck, shoulders, and jaw. The pain is not associated with nausea, vomiting, or sensitivity to light or sound. Exercise will not worsen a tension headache and may often help to relieve it. Most people with tension headaches do not seek medical treatment because the pain does not inhibit them from carrying out their normal activities, although they are occasionally severe enough to interfere with sleep. If you have a disabling headache and have been given a diagnosis of tension headache, you most likely have migraine, which almost always causes disability. Tension headaches can be episodic or chronic. Nearly everyone has experienced an occasional episodic tension headache. Episodic implies that the headaches occur less than fifteen days a month. Chronic tension headaches occur more than fifteen days a month for at least six months. Often this group has superimposed more severe migraine-like headaches that can be quite disabling.

There are approximately 25 million American *"migraineurs"* (sufferers of migraine headache), and only about half are diagnosed properly. There are three times as many women (about 18 percent of the population) as men (6 percent), most of whom are from twenty to fifty years of age. The typical age of onset is before age thirty-five, and it is unusual for migraine to start after the age of forty. Migraine attacks usually subside with age, with the incidence in postmenopausal women significantly less than in younger women. Reliable statistics are not available on how many children actually get migraines, but estimates for prepubescents range between 3 and 10 percent. Before puberty, boys and girls get migraines in roughly equal proportions, and after puberty, it is roughly the same 3:1 ratio as found in adults. Migraine has a profound economic impact in the workplace. Approximately 90 percent of migraineurs work about six days a month at half their usual level of productivity, and about 50 percent miss an average of 2.2 workdays a month. An estimated $18 billion per year is lost in decreased productivity in American female migraineurs. Migraine takes a large toll on personal and family life. Spouses and children are profoundly affected. Migraineurs miss approximately eight days of family time per year and have another twelve days of restricted activity in their personal life. Often migraines occur during a stress letdown time on weekends or on vacations, which can also greatly interfere with family life. Many migraine sufferers are often reluctant to plan family or social events for fear of developing an incapacitating migraine.

An established pattern of recurrent disabling headache is most likely migraine. Usually the pain is unilateral (one side of the head; the word *migraine* comes from the Greek word for "half the skull") and throbbing. It is associated with nausea, vomiting, and sensitivity to light and sound. The pain can be aggravated by physical activity, such as bending, climbing stairs, running, sneezing, or coughing, and usually the sufferer prefers lying down in a quiet dark room. Migraine attacks can last from 4 to 72 hours (most often between 12 and 24 hours) and usually cause moderate to severe disability. Of persons with debilitating migraine, about 40 percent endure at least one attack per month. Migraineurs often have difficulty concentrating and thinking during their attacks, limiting their ability to function. About 15 to 20 percent experience an *aura*—typically, visual disturbances, such as flashing lights, zigzag lines, or blind spots preceding the onset of pain. Less commonly, an aura can consist of tingling in an arm or leg, or even numbness or one-sided weakness. The aura usually lasts for less than one hour, comes on within an hour before the pain, and resolves when the headache symptoms begin. In addition, many migraineurs experience a prodrome or symptom complex hours to one to two days before the onset of headache, consisting of vague symptoms of fatigue, irritability, yawning, or hyperactivity. Following the resolution of pain there is frequently a feeling of lethargy or fatigue that can last for 12 to 24 hours. The symptoms in children tend to be more systemic, with nausea, vertigo, and abdominal pain often more severe than the headache.

Although **cluster** headache is much less common than migraine or tension headache, it can be much more debilitating and is often called the "suicide headache" because it is so severe. Not infrequently, sufferers of cluster headache are seen writhing in pain on the floor, pacing back and forth, or hitting their head against the wall. These headaches afflict men much more than women, in an 8:1 ratio. They usually begin in midlife, after the age of forty. They can occur in cycles with a daily headache for weeks or months at a time, followed by a headache-free period for months or even years. The headaches are usually shorter in duration than migraine, lasting approximately 45 minutes, and can occur several times per day, often at the same time each day. Not infrequently, the sufferer is awakened an hour and a half after going to sleep, since cluster headaches often begin during REM (rapid-eye-movement) sleep. These headaches are always on one side of the head, usually behind or around the eye, and accompanied by symptoms of overactivity of the parasympathetic nervous system. These might include a unilateral (on the painful side) red, tearing eye, or a runny and stuffy nostril on the painful side. About 20 percent of these people will also experience constriction of the pupil and drooping of the eyelid. The word *cluster* is used because these attacks occur daily for several weeks followed by months to years of being pain-free. Ten percent of the time clusters can become chronic, with minimal time between cycles.

CAUSES AND TRIGGERS OF HEADACHE

Tension Headache

Tension headaches used to be called muscle contraction headaches because they were thought to be caused by sustained tightness of the muscles surrounding the skull, neck, and shoulders, triggered by emotional stress and/or poor posture. However, electromyographic (EMG) measurements on both migraine and tension headache sufferers show that those with migraine have more muscle contraction of the pericranial muscles than those with tension headache. The term "muscle contraction" was replaced by "tension" because of these findings. Researchers believe that the cause of tension headache is related to the same cause as migraine but in a much milder form. Many headache specialists now believe there is a "headache continuum," with episodic tension headache on one end and migraine on the other end. In the middle of this continuum are "migrainous" headaches, which have qualities of both tension and migraine headaches. Serotonin, an important brain neurotransmitter and a critical factor in causing migraine, is also low in chronic tension headache sufferers. Although still controversial, tension headaches are now thought to be associated with changes within the neurons (nerve cells) of the brain itself, causing abnormal sensitivity to pain transmission. Another theory is that the pain results from the entrapment of substance P (a pain-related neurotransmitter) in contracted, tense muscles.

The most common *trigger* of tension headache is emotional stress. Usually the headache will come on during the stressful time, whereas migraine usually begins during the letdown time after a stressful period is over. Lack of sleep, fatigue, depression, poor nutrition, and dehydration are also common triggers. Poor posture is a very common trigger, especially associated with poor ergonomics in the workplace—e.g., prolonged typing. Spending long hours in front of a computer with poor posture can cause neck and shoulder strain, which can often trigger a headache. Another less common trigger is temporomandibular joint (TMJ) dysfunction. This can be associated with jaw pain, jaw popping, or jaw grinding (bruxism). About 40 percent of people with tension headaches have a family history of someone else with the same problem, suggesting a genetic hereditary factor. The more common *causes* and *triggers* of tension headache include:

Emotional stress, especially anxiety and depression
Poor posture
Muscle tension
Fatigue, lack of sleep, and overwork syndrome
Analgesic rebound
Lack of exercise
Eyestrain
Sinus problems
Dental problems, especially root canal treatment
TMJ (temporomandibular joint) dysfunction
Neck problems

Hypothyroidism and low adrenal function
PMS (premenstrual syndrome)
Artificial sweeteners (especially aspartame)
Alcohol
Carbon monoxide exposure
Air pollutants

Migraine Headache

The underlying cause and the pathophysiology of migraine is not completely understood. A migraine attack is thought to begin with a neurologic dysfunction in the midbrain that activates the pain sensors in the trigeminal system. (The trigeminal nerve is one of the major nerves in the head.) When the trigeminal fibers are activated, they begin a cascade of deleterious effects on the blood vessels of the meninges (the protective membrane that surrounds the brain). These include (1) dilation and release of inflammatory peptides (protein fragments), resulting in (2) inflammation of the meningeal blood vessels. This vasodilation and inflammation cause the transmission of pain back through the trigeminal nerve to the brainstem (the lower brain) and then up through the higher brain centers to the cortex, where the pain is perceived. The activation of the brainstem probably causes the associated migraine symptoms of nausea, vomiting, and sensitivity to light (photophobia), sound (phonophobia), and smell. There is also release of serotonin during a migraine, which contributes significantly to the cycle of pain-producing events with migraine. (Migraineurs typically have low levels of serotonin, even when they are pain-free.) Serotonin, a neurotransmitter with multiple functions, is stored primarily in platelets (a blood-clotting factor). The acute depletion of serotonin probably enhances the transmission of pain, although the exact mechanism is unclear. It is has been shown that an unusually high percentage of migraineurs have mitral valve prolapse, a condition that theoretically could damage platelets as they traverse the mitral valve, thus triggering the release of serotonin. The longer a migraine persists without being adequately suppressed, the more transmission there is through the higher brain centers and the more difficult it is to abort the headache. Treatment is thus directed at interrupting the pain-producing cycle of physiologic events I've just described.

Risk factors and triggers for migraine (those in *italics* are most common triggers):

Genetics—about 70 percent of migraineurs have a family history of migraine

Sleep—irregular sleep patterns, including either lack of sleep or oversleeping

Fatigue and *exhaustion*

Diet—hypoglycemia (hunger or *skipping a meal* is a common trigger, and therefore it is recommended that migraineurs eat regularly) and *food allergy,* including high *tyramine-containing foods* such as ripened *cheeses,* aged meat and fish, alcoholic beverages, certain vegetables, overripe bananas, overripe avocados (guacamole), and some fermented foods that can be headache triggers. Other "allergic" foods that most frequently cause migraine are cow's milk, wheat, corn, orange, egg, beef, yeast, tea, coffee, cane sugar, chocolate, mushrooms, and peas. There is some controversy over whether chocolate triggers migraine. It may be that some migraineurs crave chocolate as part of their prodrome. Caffeine can also be a trigger, but it is a double-edged sword. If used occasionally it can constrict the dilated blood vessels and help in aborting a migraine. This is why it is found in many headache medications, such as Excedrin, caffergot, and fiorinal. However, if you consume caffeine on a daily basis you can develop *caffeine rebound headaches,* which occur daily and can be debilitating. The most common migraine-triggering alcoholic beverages include red wine, beer, champagne, and sherry. Many migraineurs can drink white but not red wine. There are also foods that can dilate blood vessels and precipitate a migraine. These include *MSG* (monosodium glutamate), which may not be labeled as MSG and is often identified on food labels as "hydrolyzed vegetable protein" or "natural flavor" or "natural seasoning."

Although commonly known to be in Chinese food, MSG is also present in many canned, frozen, and prepackaged foods. Nutrasweet (aspartame) can also be a headache trigger. Nitrites found in hot dogs, turkey dogs, chicken dogs, and bacon are also triggers. Other foods that can cause headaches include peanuts, raw garlic, and raw onions. (Refer to the Headache Relief Diet, page 96.)

Stress—the most common trigger for migraines, usually involves *time pressure, anger,* or *worry.* Headaches often occur *after* a stressful situation, called letdown stress, such as on a weekend or the first day of a vacation. Depression, bipolar disorder, panic attacks, and generalized *anxiety* are often associated with migraine. Although there is no specific migraine personality, migraineurs tend to set high goals and spend much of their time in service to others, leaving little time for self-nurturance. They often overextend themselves by trying to achieve unrealistic goals. This leads to disappointment, fatigue, and exhaustion, which often trigger the migraines.

Hormonal factors—Many women experience menstrual migraines, occurring just before or during the menstrual period. These are often quite prolonged and debilitating. Migraines can be exacerbated by hormone replacement therapy and birth control pills, although most women can take low-estrogen oral contraceptives safely. Women who smoke, have hypertension, prolonged or complicated aura, or other neurologic symptoms associated with their migraines have an increased risk of stroke and therefore should avoid oral contraceptives as well as stopping smoking. Migraines often improve during the second and third trimester of pregnancy but often resume shortly after childbirth. Migraines can also worsen during the perimenopause and often improve with estrogen replacement. Many women experience loss of their migraines in their postmenopausal years, but some will maintain their migraines throughout their life.

Magnesium deficiency—Certain situations that can trigger migraine, such as pregnancy, use of diuretics, and drinking alcohol, are also associated with loss of magnesium. Most of the drugs used to prevent or treat migraine have some of the same physiological effects as magnesium. Magnesium levels have been shown to be low during a migraine attack.

Exertion—Regular aerobic exercise helps prevent migraines, but overexertion, dehydration, excessive sun exposure, and overheating can trigger migraine. It is important to gradually warm up and cool down as well as keep yourself well hydrated while exercising. Wearing ultraviolet protective sunglasses and a hat in the sun can also be helpful.

Rebound from withdrawal of analgesics

Cluster Headache

The cause of cluster headaches is not well understood. Just as in migraine and tension headaches, serotonin imbalance plays a significant role. There seems to be a basic malfunction in the cluster headache sufferer's biological clock, the hypothalamus, which explains why cluster headaches often strike at the same time every day or night during a cluster cycle. There is also blood vessel dilation in the carotid artery near the eye, causing the severe pain. Cluster headaches are associated with hyperstimulation of the parasympathetic nervous system, which causes the one-sided runny nose, eye tearing, pupil constriction (miosis), and eyelid drooping. Some researchers suspect that cluster headaches may be caused by a disorder in histamine metabolism, since they are usually accompanied by allergy symptoms such as tearing, nasal congestion, and a runny nose.

The most common *trigger* is alcohol. During a cluster cycle even a few drops of alcohol can trigger a severe headache. However, when not in a cluster cycle, alcohol will not trigger a headache. There is a high incidence of smoking in cluster patients, but it is not clear that this is causative or that smoking reduces the incidence of cluster headaches. Sometimes letdown stress can trigger a cluster headache, but this association is not as strong as in migraine. Unlike migraine and tension, there is no hereditary or genetic factor in cluster headaches.

LIFE-THREATENING AND OTHER TYPES OF HEADACHE

Every person who experiences recurrent headaches should be evaluated by a physician or other comparable health care provider to determine the correct diagnosis and to rule out a potentially life-threatening cause of headache. Fortunately, the following causes of headache are quite rare compared to the three types that we have focused on in this book, and are usually the ones that headache sufferers fear most. If your headaches are accompanied by double vision, projectile vomiting, weakness, paralysis, vertigo, or one-sided deafness, you should seek medical attention immediately.

Brain Tumor—The headache of a tumor is usually associated with focal neurological symptoms such as weakness of an arm or a leg, or problems with vision, coordination, speech, or memory. It can often awaken you at night, and is frequently worse upon awakening and with straining at a bowel movement, coughing, or sneezing. The best diagnostic test is an MRI brain scan.

Meningitis—This is a life-threatening infection of the covering of the brain (meninges). The three major symptoms are headache, fever, and a stiff neck. The correct diagnosis has to be made quickly and is best done with a lumbar puncture ("spinal tap") probing for evidence of bacterial infection. Once the diagnosis is made, high-dose antibiotics are given.

Subarachnoid Hemorrhage—This is usually caused by a rupture of a brain aneurysm, which is a weakening of a blood vessel in the brain. The headache comes on very suddenly and is usually the most severe pain of all headaches. The diagnosis is usually made by CAT scan and sometimes a lumbar puncture.

Stroke—The headache is usually mild and associated with focal neurologic symptoms similar to the ones seen with brain tumors. The best way to diagnose a stroke is by CAT or MRI scans.

Temporal Arteritis—This is a rare cause of headache that almost always occurs after the age of fifty and is usually associated with tenderness over the temporal arteries, which are located in the temples. They are best diagnosed by an elevated blood test called an ESR (erythrocyte sedimentation rate).

Acute Sinusitis—This is a headache caused by an infection of the sinuses and is associated with thick green or yellow postnasal or nasal mucus discharge or tenderness over the infected sinus. The definitive diagnostic test is a CAT scan of the sinuses.

Glaucoma—A rare cause of headache, this is a result of elevated eye pressure. Everyone over the age of forty should have their pressures checked, especially if there is a family history of glaucoma.

Eyestrain—This is a type of tension headache located behind the eyes that usually occurs after reading. A change in eye corrective lenses can cure this headache.

Post-traumatic—A headache can often occur after an accident that injures the neck, as in a whiplash injury incurred in a motor vehicle accident. There may not be any associated injury to the head. This headache usually comes on hours or a few days after the accident. It usually improves after several days to weeks, but can become chronic and last for months to years. The headache can have qualities of both tension and migraine and is often associated with neck and shoulder pain and stiffness. There may also be other associated debilitating symptoms, such as poor concentration, decreased ability to think about complex concepts, dizziness, depression, mood changes, decreased libido, insomnia, memory impairment, feelings of anger and frustration, lack of motivation, and irritability. This symptom complex is known as *postconcussive* syndrome. Diagnostic tests such as MRIs and blood tests are usually normal. Neuropsychological testing is the best diagnostic test to evaluate the symptoms associated with memory and cognition. Many of the treatments available for migraine and tension headaches are helpful in treating post-traumatic headaches. Trigger point injections can be helpful in treating headaches caused by problems with the neck (cervicogenic headaches). Physical therapy, proper posture, neck exercises, and yoga are also helpful.

DIAGNOSIS

Seymour Diamond, M.D., a pioneer in the treatment of migraine and director of Chicago's Diamond Headache Clinic, has recently called migraineurs "probably the most misunderstood, misdiagnosed, and mistreated group of patients in modern medicine." According to researchers addressing the 1997 World Congress of Neurology in Buenos Aires, of the 20 percent of women in the industrialized world who suffer from migraine, 40 percent are incorrectly diagnosed. And of the 5 percent of the world's male population with migraine, 80 percent are misdiagnosed, largely because migraine is commonly considered to be a condition restricted to women. Yet a skilled medical clinician can make an accurate diagnosis of tension, migraine, or cluster headache almost 90 percent of the time *through taking a complete medical history.* Most of the time it is not necessary to have a CAT scan or MRI. However, these tests can be quite helpful in ruling out other significant and possibly life-threatening causes of headache, such as those mentioned above, if any of these conditions are suspected following a thorough evaluation, including a physical and careful neurologic examination. These are often patients who present with stories not typical of migraine, tension, or cluster, such as the person who experiences a severe headache without any identifiable cause and with no previous history of headache. *A disabling recurrent headache that is stable over time is most likely migraine.*

Blood tests can help to rule out other less common systemic causes of headache, such as anemia, thyroid disease, and systemic lupus erythematosis. For example, patients with temporal arteritis have an elevated erythrocyte sedimentation rate (ESR). But it is still difficult to make a definitive diagnosis. All pain is subjective, but unlike many other painful ailments there is no blood test for migraine, tension, or cluster headaches. Many people who have been diagnosed with tension headaches actually have migraine. Remember that tension headaches are not disabling, whereas migraine interferes with your everyday activities. And many who believe they have chronic "sinus headaches" are in fact migraineurs. The typical person with chronic sinusitis has symptoms of head or nasal congestion, postnasal drainage, diminished sense of smell, yellow/green mucus drainage, and a history of sinus "problems" or infections. Sinus headaches are not as disabling as migraine. A CAT scan of the sinuses will usually show significant abnormalities within the sinuses in true sinus headache sufferers, but is usually normal in migraineurs. Although it runs in families, a specific gene has been found for only one very rare type of migraine (familial hemiplegic migraine). Migraine does show up on a PET scan (a type of brain scan)—but only if the patient can be rushed into a machine just as she's having an attack.

Most physicians also fail to diagnose migraine in those patients who do not have an aura, who make up 80 to 85 percent of migraineurs. Ninan Mathew, M.D., director of the Houston Headache Clinic, recommends not labeling a first attack as migraine. If there's not a previous history of similar episodes, he suggests waiting for repeat occurrences—five without aura or two with aura—before making the diagnosis. I would guess that if your doctor also waited that long before beginning treatment, it is most unlikely that you'd ever return to see him or her. At the present time only about 50 percent of migraineurs are being properly diagnosed, suggesting the need for increased awareness of both patients and health care providers. The following Midas (Migraine Disability Assessment) Questionnaire can help you to determine your degree of disability and to heighten your awareness of the extent to which migraines affect your life.

MIDAS QUESTIONNAIRE

Migraine Disability Assessment
(Please fill out and give to your doctor.)

Patient Name   Month/Day/Year

This questionnaire is used to determine the level of pain and disability caused by your headaches and helps your doctor find the best treatment for you.

INSTRUCTIONS: Please answer the following questions about all your headaches over the last **3 months.** Write your answer on the line next to each question. Write zero if you did not do the activity in the last **3 months.**

1. On how many days in the last 3 months did you miss work or school because of your headaches? (*If you do not attend work or school enter zero.*)   DAYS ____

2. How many days in the last 3 months was your productivity at work or school reduced by half or more because of your headaches? (*Do not include days you counted in question 1 where you missed work or school. If you do not attend school or work enter zero.*)   DAYS ____

3. On how many days in the last 3 months did you not do household work because of your headaches?   DAYS ____

4. How many days in the last 3 months was your productivity in household work reduced by half or more because of your headaches? (*Do not include days counted in question 3, where you did not do household work.*)   DAYS ____

5. On how many days in the last 3 months did you
miss family, social, or leisure activities because of
your headaches?   DAYS ____

(Questions 1–5) TOTAL ____

A. On how many days in the last 3 months did you
have a headache? (*If headache lasted more than 1 day,
count each day.*)   DAYS ____
B. On a scale of 0–10, on average, how painful were
these headaches? (*Where 0 = no pain at all, and
10 = pain which is as bad as it can be.*)   0–10 ____

After you have filled out this questionnaire, add the total number of
days from questions 1 to 5 (ignore A and B).

MIDAS GRADE	DEFINITION	MIDAS SCORE
I	Little or no disability	0–5
II	Mild disability	6–10
III	Moderate disability	11–20
IV	Severe disability	21+

CONVENTIONAL MEDICAL TREATMENT

Tension Headache

Most people with common tension headache usually do not
seek treatment because they respond to stress reduction, simple
analgesics, or sleep. A wide range of *nonprescription* analgesics is
available to treat most tension headaches. They contain either
acetaminophen 325–500 mg (Tylenol), aspirin 325 mg (Bufferin,
Empirin, Bayer), ibuprofen 200–800 mg (Advil, Nuprin,
Motrin), naproxen 250–500 mg (Naprosyn), salsalate 500 or 750
mg (Disalcid), or combinations of these ingredients: Aspirin
Free Excedrin (acetaminophen 500 mg and caffeine 65 mg) and
Extra Strength Excedrin (acetaminophen 250 mg, aspirin 250
mg, and caffeine 65 mg).

There are a number of *prescription* analgesics that are used for
treating all three types of headache. They include (in approxi-
mate order of analgesic strength):

- Phrenilin—acetaminophen 325 mg, butalbital 50 mg
- Esgic, Fioricet—acetaminophen 325 mg, caffeine 40 mg, butalbital 50 mg
- Fioricet with Codeine—acetaminophen 325 mg, caffeine 40 mg, butalbital 50 mg, codeine phosphate 30 mg
- Fiorinal—aspirin 325 mg, caffeine 40 mg, butalbital 50 mg
- Fiorinal with Codeine—aspirin 325 mg, caffeine 40 mg, butalbital 50 mg, codeine phosphate 30 mg
- Norgesic—orphenadrine citrate 25 mg, aspirin 385 mg, caffeine 30 mg
- Midrin—acetaminophen 325 mg, dichloralphenazone 100 mg, isometheptene mucate 65 mg
- Darvocet-N 50—propoxyphene napsylate 50 mg, acetaminophen 325 mg
- Darvocet-N 100—propoxyphene napsylate 100 mg, acetaminophen 650 mg
- Darvon Compound-65—propoxyphene hydrochloride 65 mg, aspirin 389 mg, caffeine 32.4 mg
- Vicodin—hydrocodone bitartrate 5 mg, acetaminophen 500 mg
- Percocet—oxycodone hydrochloride 5 mg, acetaminophen 500 mg
- Percodan—oxycodone hydrochloride 4.5 mg, oxycodone terephthalate 0.38 mg, aspirin 325 mg
- Demerol—meperidine hydrochloride 100 mg/ml injection; 50 or 100 mg tablets
- Dilaudid—hydromorphone hydrochloride 1, 2, or 4 mg/ml injection; 2 or 4 mg tablets
- Stadol—butorphanol tartrate, 1 or 2 mg/ml injection or 10 mg/ml inhalation nasal spray (spray to be used not more than twice per week.)

Conventional medical treatment for **migraine** combines the identification and elimination (if possible) of headache triggers with the use of medications to treat and prevent the pain of migraine. Prescriptions written for migraine include drugs from a number of classes, including narcotics, antidepressants, vasoconstrictors, beta-blockers, muscle relaxants, and 5-hydroxytryptophan agonists (triptans). To treat isolated mild to moderate migraine attacks, an analgesic together with an antinauseant (Phenergan, Compazine, or Reglan) may be adequate. Extra Strength Excedrin has been recommended by an FDA advisory panel for nonprescription treatment of migraine. Combination prescription medications, including opiates, barbiturates, and codeine-containing drugs, can be sparingly used as rescue medications for moderate to severe headaches but should be monitored very carefully because of risk of abuse. It is important to avoid using any of the prescription analgesics and combination drugs on the above list for more than two days a week, since migraineurs can transform from having intermittent episodic headaches to chronic daily debilitating headaches due to excessive use of analgesics (analgesic rebound). These patients have to be detoxed off these daily medications in order for effective treatment to take place. The more severe and disabling migraine attacks require drugs that are more specific for migraine, such as *ergot* preparations or one of the *triptans.*

The ergotamines (Ergomar, Wigraine) are the most commonly used class of drugs in treating acute migraine. After earlier research (in the 1970s) concluded that the dilating of the blood vessels surrounding the brain was the precipitating event in migraine, treatment relied on reversing the dilation with drugs that caused the vessels to constrict. Those that were most effective were compounds derived from the rye fungus ergot. Formulations containing ergotamine are now well established in treating acute migraine. The more commonly prescribed ergotamine medications are Cafergot and Wigraine (both oral tablets and suppositories), Ergostat and Ergomar (sublingual tablets), Bellergal-S (oral tablets), and Migranal (nasal spray). They are often accompanied by an antinauseant. But ergotamine is a powerful vasoconstrictor and ergot drugs have side effects that many patients cannot tolerate. These include paresthesias (tingling of hands or feet), muscle cramps, claudication (tension and weakness of hands or feet), and coldness of fingers or toes. In rare cases it can even result in gangrene of the fingers or toes. Ergot drugs are contraindicated in people with peripheral vascular disease, coronary artery disease, thrombophlebitis, or hypertension, as well as in pregnant or lactating women and in the very old.

Oral ergotamine is easy to use but can produce nausea and may be poorly absorbed. Sublingual tablets are more rapidly absorbed but may also cause nausea. Also well absorbed and with less nausea are the suppositories. In 1997 Migranal first became available and, as a nasal spray, is the fastest way to deliver ergot to the brain. But not all patients respond to ergotamine, and some who do become habituated use them daily and wake up every day with a "rebound" headache that is almost as bad as the migraine it's replacing.

Imitrex (sumatriptan), introduced in 1993, is still the most widely used medication for treating migraine. It was joined in the late 1990s by the other *triptans*—Zomig (zolmitriptan), Amerge (naratriptan), and Maxalt (rizotriptan)—and together these drugs have "changed the whole face of treating migraine," according to Alan Rapoport, M.D., director of the New England Center for Headache in Stamford, Connecticut. They relieve migraine by inhibiting pain transmission from peripheral branches of the trigeminal nerve in the meningeal blood vessels surrounding the brain. They're serotonin agonists, which means that their method of action is to stimulate the serotonin receptors in these blood vessels (this increases uptake of serotonin), thus causing vasoconstriction along with inhibition of the release of pain-producing inflammatory neuropeptides, thereby controlling the source of pain in migraine. Unlike Imitrex, the newer triptans cross the blood-brain barrier and act on the receptors of the trigeminal nerve located in the brain stem and provide an additional block to the central transmission of the pain in migraine. They work faster and last longer than Imitrex.

All triptans, however, are cleared from the body in a few hours, and the migraine sometimes returns. Some physicians will prescribe different triptans and different modes of administration (oral or injectable) for various degrees of headache. Imitrex is available in subcutaneous (just under the skin) injectable form (these can be self-administered), oral (25 and 50 mg tablets), and nasal spray. Following an injection, relief of headache and associated symptoms (nausea, photophobia, etc.) usually occurs in 10 to 30 minutes. If relief is not obtained, a second dose may be given after 1 hour. The maximum recommended dosage is two injections in 24 hours, separated by at least 1 hour. For oral Imitrex, the recommended initial dose is 25 or 50 mg. If necessary, a second dose may be given 2 hours later. Additional oral doses may be taken at intervals of at least 2 hours, up to a maximum of 300 mg/day. One study evaluating its effectiveness revealed that 2 hours after taking an initial dose of 50 mg orally, 61 percent of patients improved significantly and 31 percent were pain-free. Imitrex works even faster when taken by nasal spray or injection. The newer triptans are available only in oral form.

There are still many people for whom Imitrex and the triptans don't work, in addition to those who cannot tolerate the side effects or are not candidates for these drugs. Common side effects include tightness or pressure in the chest and neck, occasional difficulty breathing, facial flushing, and a "rush" sensation to the head. The triptans are vasoconstrictors and are contraindicated in people with coronary artery disease (e.g., angina or a previous heart attack), uncontrolled hypertension, prior stroke, hemiplegic/basilar migraine, or seizures/epilepsy, and in pregnant women. They should not be combined with ergotamine. Particular caution should also be exercised when these drugs are first used in people who may be at risk for unrecognized coronary artery disease (e.g., postmenopausal women, heavy smokers, or someone with hypercholesterolemia, obesity, diabetes, or a strong family history of coronary disease).

The treatment of migraine in pregnancy poses a bit of a challenge because most antimigraine drugs cross the placental barrier and can damage the fetus. Acetaminophen is considered safe but is only mildly effective, while aspirin, ergot, and the triptans are all contraindicated. Demerol may be considered as a last resort for severe headache relief if its use is carefully regulated. Migraines usually diminish in the last two trimesters of pregnancy.

Depression can also complicate migraine. Increased risk of suicide has been reported in people with depression and migraine with aura. Prozac and Elavil have dual effects on depression and migraine and can be quite helpful when both conditions are present. Depakote is effective for people with migraine and bipolar disorders, as well as those with panic disorder and migraine. Benzodiazepines (Valium, Xanax) are not recommended for this latter group because of the risks of habituation and dependence with prolonged use.

The decision to use daily preventive medication for migraine is based on the frequency, duration, and intensity of the attacks. Prophylactic medications are usually considered in patients who have two or three disabling migraines or one prolonged attack per month. Other candidates are patients who have poor responses to acute therapy and those in whom acute agents are contraindicated. The preventive drugs most commonly used include:

- beta-blockers—Nadolol, Inderal, Tenormin, Blocadren
- calcium channel blockers—Calan SR, Isoptin SR, Adalat, Procardia, Cardizem, Nimotop
- tricyclic antidepressants—Elavil, Pamelor, Tofranil, Norpramin, Apapin, Sinequan, Desyrel, Prozac
- anticonvulsants—Depakote, Neurontin
- serotonin antagonist—Sansert

Each of these groups of drugs has significant side effects that must be considered before the decision is made to begin preventive therapy. Prophylactic medications at appropriately reduced dosages are indicated if migraine attacks are frequent—i.e., at least two per month—and severe. Periactin in a dosage of 4 to 6 mg/day has been shown to be effective in children in one controlled study, while several studies have demonstrated the benefits of behavioral therapy in preventing chronic migraine in children.

Cluster headache is perhaps the most difficult to treat. Multiple medications are often required and a strong focus on prevention is needed. Sublingual ergotamine may be given at onset and repeated once if necessary. Dihydroergotamine (DHE) 1 mg is also effective. DHE is chemically similar to ergotamine, but it has less vasoconstrictive action, which makes it safer than ergotamine. It is available only in injectable form. Subcutaneous Imitrex is useful, but, because of the recurrent nature of cluster headaches, it may have to be given in doses that exceed those recommended for adequate headache control. Lidocaine nasal spray can also be effective. Cluster headache can often be successfully treated with inhalation of 100% oxygen by face mask at a rate of 7 liters/minute for 15 to 20 minutes, with the patient seated and leaning forward. This can be repeated as needed after a 5-minute rest.

For prevention of cluster headache, patients are advised to avoid smoking, alcohol, and exposure to triggers such as nitrites, strong perfumes, volatile solvents, and gasoline fumes, during their cluster cycles. Highly stressful situations and high-pressure tasks should also be avoided. If the headaches are usually associated with a letdown period, stress-management techniques can also be helpful. Cluster headache attacks may occur at high altitudes with low oxygen levels during air travel. Ergotamine 2 mg, taken 1 hour before takeoff, may prevent these attacks. If a headache does occur during flight, inhalation from the passenger's overhead oxygen supply may abort it. Prophylactic medications for cluster headache include verapimil 120 to 480 mg/day; prednisone 60 mg/day to start, then tapered over 3 weeks; lithium 300 to 900 mg/day; and Depakote 600 to 2,000 mg/day. A reduced dose of lithium is required if calcium channel blockers or NSAIDs are used concurrently. Lithium has added value in patients who are also suffering from manic episodes of bipolar disorder.

Chapter 3

HOLISTIC HEALTH:
THE THRIVING SELF-TEST

The only thing I know that truly heals people is unconditional love.
—ELISABETH KÜBLER-ROSS, M.D.

Most people who read this book have recurrent and probably severe headaches and may not consider themselves to be particularly healthy. But **what is health?** The conditioning that the majority of us have grown up with has taught us to define health as the absence of illness. We may respond to the question "Are you healthy?" by thinking, *I'm not sick, so I must be healthy.* Yet the words *health, heal,* and *holy* are all derived from the same Old English word, *haelan,* which means "to make whole." Viewed from this perspective, two questions that more directly and accurately address the issue of health are "Do you love your life?" and "Are you happy to be alive?" For health is far more than simply a matter of not feeling ill: It is the daily experience of *wholeness and balance—a state of being fully alive in body, mind, and spirit.* Such a condition could also be called optimal, or holistic health, or wellness. I call it *thriving.* Helping you to achieve this state of total well-being is the primary objective of this book. *As a by-product of that enlivening process, your headaches will either improve significantly or be cured.*

HALLMARKS OF OPTIMAL HEALTH

Optimal health results from harmony and balance in the physical, environmental, mental, emotional, spiritual, and social aspects of our lives. When this harmonious balance is present, we experience the *unlimited and unimpeded free flow of life-force energy throughout our body, mind, and spirit.* Around the world, this energy is known by many names. The Chinese call it *qi* ("chee"), the Japanese refer to it as *ki,* in India it is known as *prana,* and in Hebrew it is *chai.* But in the Western world, the phrase that comes closest to capturing the feeling generated by this energy is *unconditional love,* regarded by holistic physicians as *our most powerful healer.*

Although each of us has the capacity to nurture and to heal ourselves, most of us have yet to tap into this wellspring of loving life energy. Yet there is no one who can better administer this life-enhancing elixir to you than you yourself.

By committing to caring for yourself in the manner recommended in the following chapters, you will in essence be learning how to better *give and receive love*—to yourself and others. As a result, you will be enhancing the flow of life-force energy throughout every aspect of your life. This holistic healing process will also provide you with the opportunity to safely and effectively treat your headache and any other physical, mental, and spiritual conditions that may be impeding the flow of healing energy in your life.

Living a holistically healthy lifestyle can facilitate the realization of your ideal life vision in accordance with both your personal and professional goals. But since the majority of us are only aware of health as a condition of not being sick, a mental image of what living holistically means is needed in order to achieve it. Briefly, let's examine this state of optimal well-being to give you a glimpse of what it looks and feels like.

A list of the six components of health follows, the first italicized item in each category encompassing the essence of that component. For example, physical health can be simply described as a condition of *high energy and vitality,* while mental health is a state of *peace of mind and contentment.* The italicized items can also serve as a health gauge you can use to measure your progress in each area.

PHYSICAL HEALTH
High energy and vitality
- Freedom from, or high adaptability to, pain, dysfunction, and disability
- A strong immune system
- A body that feels light, balanced, strong, flexible, and has good aerobic capacity
- Ability to meet physical challenges and perform exceptionally
- Full capacity of all five senses and a healthy libido

ENVIRONMENTAL HEALTH
Harmony with your environment (neither harming nor being harmed)
- Awareness of your connectedness with nature
- Feeling grounded—comfort and security within your surroundings
- Respect and appreciation for your home, the earth, and all of her inhabitants
- Contact with the earth; breathing healthy air; drinking pure water; eating uncontaminated food; exposure to the sun, fire, or candlelight; immersion in warm water (all on a daily basis)

MENTAL HEALTH
Peace of mind and contentment
- A job that you love doing
- Optimism
- A sense of humor
- Financial well-being
- Living your life vision
- The ability to express your creativity and talents
- The capacity to make healthy decisions

EMOTIONAL HEALTH

Self-acceptance and high self-esteem
- The capacity to identify, express, experience, and accept all of your feelings, both painful and joyful
- Awareness of the intimate connection between your physical and emotional bodies
- The ability to confront your greatest fears
- The fulfillment of your capacity to play
- Peak experiences on a regular basis

SPIRITUAL HEALTH

Experience of unconditional love/absence of fear
- Soul awareness and a personal relationship with God or Spirit
- Trust in your intuition and an openness to change
- Gratitude
- Creating a sacred space on a regular basis through prayer, meditation, walking in nature, observing a Sabbath day, or other rituals
- Sense of purpose
- Being present in every moment

SOCIAL HEALTH

Intimacy with a spouse or partner, relative, or close friend
- Effective communication
- Forgiveness
- Sense of belonging to a support group or community
- Touch and/or physical intimacy on a daily basis
- Selflessness and altruism

The Thriving Self-Test

Now that you understand the six categories that constitute optimal health, it's time to measure how close you are to *thriving* in each area. The following questionnaire is designed to provide you with a much clearer idea of the status of your health in all six areas. You can use the results of the test to guide you through the rest of the book and it can become a blueprint for restructuring your life. You can also measure your progress by retaking the test every two or three months.

Answer the questions in each section below and total your score. Each response will be a number from 0 to 5. Please refer to the frequency described within the parentheses (e.g., "2 to 3 times/week") when answering questions about an *activity*—for example, "Do you maintain a healthy diet?" However, when the question refers to an *attitude* or an *emotion* (most of the Mind and Spirit questions—for example, "Do you have a sense of humor?"), the response is more subjective and less exact, and you should refer to the terms describing the frequency, such as *often* or *daily,* but not to the numbered frequencies in parentheses:

0 = Never or almost never (once a year or less)
1 = Seldom (2 to 12 times/year)
2 = Occasionally (2 to 4 times/month)
3 = Often (2 to 3 times/week)
4 = Regularly (4 to 6 times/week)
5 = Daily (every day).

Body: Physical and Environmental Health

_____ 1. Do you maintain a healthy diet (low fat, low sugar, fresh fruits, grains, and vegetables)?

_____ 2. Is your water intake adequate (at least ½ oz./lb. of body weight; 160 lbs. = 80 ounces)?

_____ 3. Are you within 20 percent of your ideal body weight?

_____ 4. Do you feel physically attractive?

_____ 5. Do you fall asleep easily and sleep soundly?

_____ 6. Do you awaken in the morning feeling well rested?

_____ 7. Do you have more than enough energy to meet your daily responsibilities?

_____ 8. Are your five senses acute?

_____ 9. Do you take time to experience sensual pleasure?

_____10. Do you schedule regular massage or deep-tissue body work?

_____11. Does your sexual relationship feel gratifying?

_____12. Do you engage in regular physical workouts (lasting at least 20 minutes)?

_____13. Do you have good endurance or aerobic capacity?

_____14. Do you breathe abdominally for at least a few minutes?

_____15. Do you maintain physically challenging goals?

_____16. Are you physically strong?

_____17. Do you do some stretching exercises?

_____18. Are you free of chronic aches, pains, ailments, and diseases?

_____19. Do you have regular effortless bowel movements?

_____20. Do you understand the causes of your chronic physical problems?

_____21. Are you free of any drug (including caffeine and nicotine) or alcohol dependency?

_____22. Do you live and work in a healthy environment with respect to clean air, water, and indoor pollution?

_____23. Do you feel energized or empowered by nature?

_____24. Do you feel a strong connection with and appreciation for your body, your home, and your environment?

_____25. Do you have an awareness of life-force energy or *qi* ("chee")?

_____ TOTAL BODY SCORE

Mind: Mental and Emotional Health

_____ 1. Do you have specific goals in your personal and professional life?

_____ 2. Do you have the ability to concentrate for extended periods of time?

_____ 3. Do you use visualization or mental imagery to help you attain your goals or enhance your performance?

_____ 4. Do you believe it is possible to change?

_____ 5. Can you meet your financial needs and desires?

_____ 6. Is your outlook basically optimistic?

_____ 7. Do you give yourself more supportive messages than critical messages?

_____ 8. Does your job utilize all of your greatest talents?

_____ 9. Is your job enjoyable and fulfilling?

_____10. Are you willing to take risks or make mistakes in order to succeed?

_____11. Are you able to adjust beliefs and attitudes as a result of learning from painful experiences?

_____12. Do you have a sense of humor?

_____13. Do you maintain peace of mind and tranquillity?

_____14. Are you free from a strong need for control or the need to be right?

_____15. Are you able to fully experience (feel) your painful feelings such as fear, anger, sadness, and hopelessness?

_____16. Are you aware of and able to safely express fear?

_____17. Are you aware of and able to safely express anger?

_____18. Are you aware of and able to safely express sadness (or cry)?

_____19. Are you accepting of all your feelings?

_____20. Do you engage in meditation, contemplation, or psychotherapy to better understand your feelings?

_____21. Is your sleep free from disturbing dreams?

_____22. Do you explore the symbolism and emotional content of your dreams?

_____23. Do you take the time to relax, or make time for activities that constitute the abandon or absorption of play?

_____24. Do you experience feelings of exhilaration?

_____25. Do you enjoy high self-esteem?

_____   TOTAL MIND SCORE

Spirit: Spiritual and Social Health

_____ 1. Do you actively commit time to your spiritual life?

_____ 2. Do you take time for prayer, meditation, or reflection?

_____ 3. Do you listen to and act upon your intuition?

_____ 4. Are creative activities a part of your work or leisure time?

_____ 5. Do you take risks?

_____ 6. Do you have faith in a God, spirit guides, or angels?

_____ 7. Are you free from anger toward God?

_____ 8. Are you grateful for the blessings in your life?

_____ 9. Do you take walks, garden, or have contact with nature?

_____10. Are you able to let go of your attachment to specific outcomes and embrace uncertainty?

_____11. Do you observe a day of rest completely away from work, dedicated to nurturing yourself and your family?

_____12. Can you let go of self-interest in deciding the best course of action for a given situation?

_____ 13. Do you feel a sense of purpose?

_____ 14. Do you make time to connect with young children, either your own or someone else's?

_____ 15. Are playfulness and humor important to you in your daily life?

_____ 16. Do you have the ability to forgive yourself and others?

_____ 17. Have you demonstrated the willingness to commit to a marriage or comparable long-term relationship?

_____ 18. Do you experience intimacy, besides sex, in your committed relationships?

_____ 19. Do you confide in or speak openly with one or more close friends?

_____ 20. Do you or did you feel close to your parents?

_____ 21. If you have experienced the loss of a loved one, have you fully grieved that loss?

_____ 22. Has your experience of pain enabled you to grow spiritually?

_____ 23. Do you go out of your way or give your time to help others?

_____ 24. Do you feel a sense of belonging to a group or community?

_____ 25. Do you experience unconditional love?

_____ TOTAL SPIRIT SCORE

_____ TOTAL BODY, MIND, SPIRIT SCORE

Health Scale:

325–375	Optimal Health: **Thriving**
275–324	Excellent Health
225–274	Good Health
175–224	Fair Health
125–174	Below Average Health
75–124	Poor Health
Less than 75	Extremely Unhealthy: **Surviving**

Once you complete this questionnaire, pay attention to which categories you need to make the most improvements in, and remember that *there are multiple factors that have combined to cause your headaches.* Then start to implement the tools and suggestions that are outlined in Chapters 4, 5, and 6. Chapter 4 gives you a blueprint for improving your physical and environmental health while also specifically addressing headaches and strengthening your immune system. Chapter 5 outlines a holistic approach for mental and emotional health, while Chapter 6 will help you enhance your spiritual and social health. Begin where you are most comfortable and take your time. You are committing to a life-changing process, one that requires patience and discipline, so proceed at your own pace. Remember, too, that everyone is unique and no two of us will follow the exact same healing path. While the science of holistic medicine provides a universal foundation and structure, its *art* lies in the writing of your own personal prescription for optimal health, so feel free to adapt the techniques in the pages ahead to tailor-make the holistic self-care program that is most ideally suited for you. Your heart will be your primary guide on this odyssey of realizing your full potential as a human being.

During the fifteen years that I've been actively engaged in this healing process, I've identified several practices that have had the deepest impact on my health, the most transformative effect upon my life, and will provide the greatest therapeutic benefits for your headaches. I call them the *essential 8 for optimal health:*

1. Air and Breathing
2. Water and Moisture
3. Food and Supplements
4. Exercise and Rest
5. Play/Passion/Purpose
6. Gratitude and Prayer
7. Intimacy
8. Forgiveness

As you read the following chapters and begin incorporating the Headache Survival Program into your life, keep these *essential 8* in mind. (I've numbered them throughout the book, 1 through 8, to help you remember.) They are the basis of this holistic treatment program and can become the structure upon which the rest of your life is built.

Chapter 4

HEALING YOUR BODY
The Physical and Environmental Health Components of the Headache Survival Program

I f you would rather not learn to live with your migraine, cluster, and tension headaches or become dependent on medications along with experiencing a diminished quality of life, then I would like to take you on a healing journey into an exciting new (yet ancient) frontier of medicine. For the past fourteen years, I have been practicing **holistic medicine** while treating headaches, arthritis, sinusitis, backache, and a variety of other so-called chronic or incurable conditions. The Headache Survival Program has its foundation in the holistic practice of treating, preventing, and potentially curing any chronic condition, as well as creating a state of optimal well-being. Although the bulk of the holistic approach is similar for any chronic condition or disease, this and the following chapters include specific dietary, nutritional supplement, herbal recommendations, professional care therapies, as well as emotional factors that relate directly to treating the *causes and symptoms* of headache. *Commitment* to this approach has resulted in a significant improvement of the symptoms of tension, migraine, and cluster headaches, in addition to a far greater experience of well-being in many people. This success stems primarily from the basic *health* orientation of the holistic approach. Rather than focusing on the disease and just treating its symptoms—they are certainly not ignored, just perceived differently—holistic medicine addresses *causes* while restoring balance and harmony to the *whole person*. It goes far beyond the "quick fix" (outlined in Chapter 1) or the repair of a "broken part," to an understanding of *what can be learned from your physical pain and how to use that knowledge to change your life and be free of headaches.*

I was led to the practice of holistic medicine and a condition of optimal health by my painful sinuses. My guide on this healing path was, and still is, Hippocrates, who recognized 2,500 years ago the most direct and effective method for training to become a healer: "Physician, heal thyself." In the remainder of this book, I'd like to guide you on a similar path leading not only to the healing of your painful head and any other dis-ease, but to a state of holistic health. By taking the Thriving Self-Test in Chapter 3, you have measured your present state of well-being. I'd recommend repeating this test every two to three months to gauge your physical, mental, and spiritual health progress and in your training as a healer of yourself.

In the process of healing your body along with your headaches, the ultimate objective is the following state of physical and environmental well-being:

PHYSICAL HEALTH
High energy and vitality
- Freedom from, or high adaptability to, pain, dysfunction, and disability
- A strong immune system
- A body that feels light, balanced, strong, flexible, and has good aerobic capacity
- Ability to meet physical challenges and perform exceptionally
- Full capacity of all five senses and a healthy libido

ENVIRONMENTAL HEALTH
Harmony with your environment (neither harming nor being harmed)
- Awareness of your connectedness with nature

- Feeling grounded—comfort and security within your surroundings
- Respect and appreciation for your home, the earth, and all of her inhabitants
- Contact with the earth; breathing healthy air; drinking pure water; eating uncontaminated food; exposure to the sun, fire, or candlelight; immersion in warm water (all on a daily basis)

HOLISTIC MEDICAL TREATMENT AND PREVENTION

To begin to restore your body to a heightened state of harmony and to correct the present imbalance manifested by headaches, your *primary goals* are:

1. **To identify and avoid each of the triggers of your headaches**
2. **To reduce inflammation and muscle tension**

In meeting these goals you can potentially cure yourself of headaches while you're healing your life. The word *cure* refers to a physical problem, while *heal* has to do with the condition of your life. However, it is possible to cure your headaches but still be living an imbalanced life; or conversely you may feel whole, balanced, at peace with your life while still experiencing some degree of pain. In essence, *this holistic approach will provide you with the potential to do both—cure headaches and heal your life—while you are engaged in the process of loving and nurturing your aching head along with the rest of you.*

Think of the Headache Survival Program as *a personalized course in self-healing and optimal well-being.* In this and the following chapters, you will be provided with a "curriculum," or, if you prefer, a "prescription," for improving six components of health, while treating each of the primary causes of headache. I have tried to simplify each component and have suggested a range of new tools to help you find your own path to a greater level of physical, environmental, mental, emotional, spiritual, and social fitness. These tools must be practiced regularly in order to be effective. (However, if, after giving it a fair trial, a particular practice feels too uncomfortable to you, then stop.) If you are willing to be patient—remember, it took years for you to develop your current state of health—I promise that you will feel better, but I cannot guarantee you will cure your headaches. However, your chances for doing so are far greater using this approach than if you strictly adhered to conventional medical treatment that focuses on using drugs to treat symptoms. Holistic medicine is not an alternative, but a complement to what you are already doing for your headaches. It is also the most therapeutically sound and cost-effective approach to the treatment of chronic ailments that I've found in nearly thirty years of practicing medicine. By taking responsibility for your own health, you become not only your own healer but a highly skilled practitioner of preventive medicine. You'll learn what *causes* your head to ache and what relieves the pain, and you will be able to make well-informed choices regarding your headache problem. You're also somewhat of a pioneer, since the holistic self-care model presented on the following pages will soon become an essential part of the foundation of primary care medicine. Keep in mind that although this is a course with a lot of homework, there are no exams or grades, no mistakes or failures—just a series of valuable lessons to help you feel more fully alive. Enjoy yourself! What do you have to lose?

SYMPTOM TREATMENT

I would recommend beginning the Headache Survival Program with an aggressive approach to treating the most uncomfortable symptoms of your headache. This includes consulting with your physician and making sure that you have treated your condition with the best methods that conventional medicine has to offer, even if they provide only temporary and symptomatic relief. It is also essential that you determine if the benefits of that treatment outweigh the liabilities. For instance, analgesics and anti-inflammatories may be harmful to the gastrointestinal tract, possibly causing stomach ulcers. Taking non-steroidal anti-inflammatories (NSAIDs) over time also accelerates cartilage loss and can contribute to osteoarthritis. (See my book *Arthritis Survival*). Liver and kidney damage is also a well-known risk for chronic use of NSAIDs. If you've decided the risks for continuing this course of symptom treatment are too great or that it's not giving you effective relief, there are several options that will be offered to you in this chapter.

As you begin the Headache Survival Program, it is helpful to rate each of your symptoms on a scale of 1 to 10, with 1 being an almost incapacitating symptom and 10 being perfectly normal (no symptom). You can use the Symptom Chart (page 56) and rate yourself at the end of each week. It provides you with both an objective (most of the symptoms can be measured objectively—you can either see, hear, or feel them) and subjective (energy level, emotions) means of monitoring your progress. You don't need anyone else or an X ray or lab test to tell you how well you're doing. Please add any symptoms to this chart that are not listed but that often cause you discomfort.

The foundation of the physical aspect of holistic medical treatment is to love and nurture your body with safe, gentle, and effective therapies. You should have a much better idea of how to do that, especially for your aching head, after reading this chapter. Remember that the essentials of the Physical Health Component of the Headache Survival Program can also be found in Chapter 1. As you begin, you should now envision your muscles letting go, melting, like butter on a hot day. See your muscles as relaxed yet toned, easily and effortlessly supporting your head atop your neck. See your head, neck, and face fully relieved of tension and pain, and your energy is perfect. This healing vision can be expanded in any way you'd like. But it is important to keep it in mind as often as you can, since it will help you to stay focused on the goal of your treatment, and even more important, to make that vision become a reality.

Symptom Chart

Began Headache Survival Program on_____.
Rate symptoms from 1 (worst) to 10 (best = normal).

SYMPTOM	BEGIN _____ (date)	END WEEK 1	END WEEK 2	END WEEK 3	END WEEK 4	END WEEK 5	END WEEK 6	END WEEK 7	END WEEK 8	END WEEK 9	END WEEK 10	END WEEK 11	END WEEK 12
Head Pain													
Jaw Pain													
Neck Pain													
Nausea													
Vomiting													
Photophobia (sensitivity to light)													
Phonophobia (sensitivity to sound or movement)													
Cognitive impairment (memory, thinking, concentration)													
Aura													
Depression													
Fatigue (energy level)													
Unilateral (one-sided) nasal congestion													
Eye tearing													
Eyelid drooping													
Eye redness													

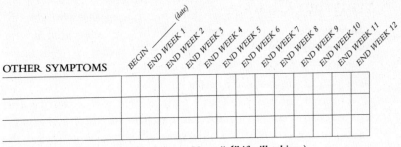

OTHER SYMPTOMS

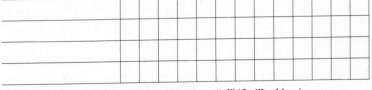

MEDICATIONS (pharmaceutical drugs: Use a "✓" if still taking.)

VITAMINS/HERBS/SUPPLEMENTS (Use a "✓" if still taking.)

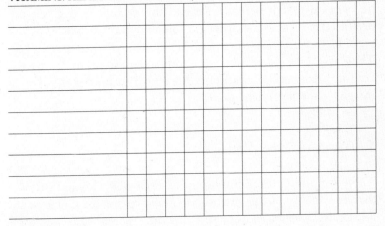

PHYSICAL AND ENVIRONMENTAL HEALTH RECOMMENDATIONS FOR HEADACHE AND OPTIMAL HEALTH

Headache, like any other chronic condition viewed from a holistic medical perspective, is a systemic dis-ease reflecting an imbalance and disharmony in the whole person—body, mind, and spirit. However, if your initial treatment is aggressively directed toward eliminating each of the triggers that you identify, while healing and restoring balance to your life—that is, improving both your mental and spiritual health as well as the physical—you have an excellent chance of curing your headaches using this holistic approach.

The first and foremost goal of treatment is to **identify and then reduce or eliminate each of the headache triggers.** In holistic medicine this objective will guide you toward the best methods for nurturing yourself in body, mind, and spirit. Use the triggers, and especially the specific emotional stressors, as messengers that will direct your healing process. Dr. Peters has developed the Headache Diary (pages 60 and 61), which he recommends to help his patients identify their headache triggers and to monitor their progress in treating them.

As I mentioned at the conclusion of Chapter 3, I've identified several practices that have had the deepest impact on my health, the most transformative effect upon my life, and will provide the greatest therapeutic benefits for your headaches. They will quickly reduce or eliminate most of the potential common triggers of headache. Air and Breathing is the first of the *essential 8 for optimal health.*

1. Air and Breathing

There is nothing more important to optimal health and survival than the quality of the air and our ability to breathe it. There are also several *environmental* factors that can trigger headaches, such as a lack of oxygen resulting from high altitude, air pollution, and carbon monoxide; a change in weather or barometric pressure; cigarette smoke and perfumes; extremely dry air; noise; sunlight glare; ion depletion or imbalance (too few negative ions, or an excess of positive ions); and extreme heat or cold. It is also possible to experience an oxygen deficiency from breathing inefficiently. In the following pages I will describe *how to avoid these environmental headache triggers while creating optimal indoor air,* and suggest several exercises for more efficient breathing.

You have already learned that sinusitis (an inflammation or infection of a sinus cavity) can be a frequent and significant cause of headaches. Both the painful swelling of the mucous membrane lining the sinuses and the subsequent congestion and obstruction of air flow can contribute to triggering headaches. It is the job of the nose and sinuses to protect the lungs. They do so by functioning as the body's:

1. air filter—they remove particles, pollen, smoke, mold, animal dander, bacteria, and viruses
2. humidifier—they moisten dry air
3. temperature regulator—they warm cold air and cool extremely hot air

If the nose and sinuses are not functioning at peak efficiency, then you may become more susceptible to several of the environmental headache triggers—air pollution, weather and barometric changes, cigarette smoke, perfumes, ion depletion, dry air, and temperature extremes. Or if they're congested or infected with allergies, a cold, or a sinus infection, then you may not be getting quite enough oxygen (another headache trigger), and the lungs are potentially at greater risk for developing asthma or bronchitis. The health of the lungs is intimately connected to that of the nose and sinuses, while the proper functioning of all three parts of the respiratory tract is helpful in preventing headaches and necessary for providing the body with an optimal supply of oxygen. The following recommendations will assist you in creating a healthy indoor environment and respiratory tract, in preventing headaches, and in experiencing optimal health.

OPTIMAL AIR QUALITY

The first step in improving both your physical and environmental health is to change the quality of the indoor air you're

Your Headache Diary*

Headache Keys

(*1) SEVERITY SCALE

(*4) RELIEF SCALE

1		5		10	1		5		10
None	Mild		Moderate	Severe	Complete	Mild	Moderate		No Relief

Date	Time Onset / Ending (Insert hour and a.m./p.m.)	(*1) Severity of headache	(*2) Psych. & physical factors	(*3) Food and drink

(*2) Psychological and physical factors

1. Emotional upset/family or friends
2. Emotional upset/occupation
3. Business/reversal
4. Pushing self too hard
5. Vacation days
6. Weekends
7. Strenuous exercise
8. Strenuous labor
9. High-altitude location
10. Anticipation anxiety
11. Crisis/serious
12. Post-crisis period

13. New job/position
14. New move
15. Menstrual days
16. Physical illness
17. Oversleeping
18. Too little sleep
19. Weather
20. Skipping meal
21. Insufficient rest and relaxation
22. Bright light or loud noise
23. Other

*Reprinted with permission from Ken Peters, M.D.

Medication taken and dosage	Non-medication approach	(*4) Relief of headache

(*3) Food and drink

A. Ripened cheeses (pizza)
B. Herring
C. Chocolate
D. Vinegar
E. Fermented foods (pickled or marinated) (sour cream/yogurt)
F. Freshly baked yeast products
G. Nuts (peanut butter)
H. Monosodium glutamate (Chinese foods)
I. Pods of broad beans
J. Raw onions or garlic
K. Canned figs
L. Citrus foods
M. Bananas
N. Pork
O. Caffeinated drinks (colas)
P. Avocados
Q. Fermented sausage (cured cold cuts)
R. Chicken livers
S. Wine
T. Alcohol
U. Beer

breathing—in essence, to create healing rather than harmful or irritating air. All of the recommendations mentioned in this section are helpful. But at the very least I would start with a negative-ion generator in your bedroom and, if you can afford it, in your workplace as well. Within three to four weeks, I would add a warm-mist humidifier in the bedroom (especially during the winter months), along with plants in the house, an effective furnace filter, followed by air duct and carpet cleaning. If the expense does not deter you, then a central humidifier installed on the furnace will complete your indoor air enhancement program. You may not create optimal indoor air, but you'll be close. Ideal air quality is rated by clarity (freedom from pollutants), humidity (between 35 and 55 percent), temperature (between 65° and 85°F), oxygen content (21 percent of total volume and 100 percent saturation), and negative ion content (3,000 to 6,000 .001-micron ions per cubic centimeter). Air that is clean, moist, warm, oxygen-rich, and high in negative ions is the healthiest air a human being can breathe.

Not only are we dependent on oxygen for survival, but every part of the human body thrives with a maximum supply of oxygen. If your respiratory tract is defective because of a nasal, sinus, or lung ailment, or if the amount of oxygen available in the air is relatively low—air that is high in carbon monoxide and/or other pollutants, air at higher altitudes (oxygen content decreases by over 3 percent every thousand feet above sea level), or stale indoor air—your body is receiving less than its optimal requirement of oxygen. Headache is often the first symptom of a lack of oxygen. Scientists report that the oxygen content of the air in some polluted cities is as low as 8 percent instead of the normal 21 percent. If you live in a polluted high-altitude city such as Denver, Salt Lake City, or Albuquerque, then your body is receiving far less oxygen than it needs for optimal function.

Negative ions are air molecules that have excess electrons. Negative ions vitalize or freshen the air we breathe by removing unhealthy particles. The earth itself is a natural negative-ion generator. Health spas have always been located in areas high in negative ions (3,000 to 20,000 per cubic centimeter of air), such

as along seacoasts, near rushing streams and waterfalls, in moun-
tainous areas, and in pine forests (pine needles cause negative ions
to be generated in the surrounding air). Although unproven,
there is speculation that negative ions increase the sweeping motion of the cilia on the respiratory mucosa, and subsequently enhance the movement of mucus and the clearing or filtering of
inhaled pollutants. Unfortunately, there is very little research on
the effect of negative ions on the respiratory tract. Two studies
were performed in the 1960s in Israel that indicated negative
ions had a beneficial effect on asthmatics, but to my knowledge
there has been no recent research. Although there is no scientific
documentation of the effect of negative ions on headaches, for
the past decade I have seen many patients who can attest to the
therapeutic benefit of breathing ion-rich air for quickly relieving headaches. What has been conclusively proven is that negative ions are effective air cleaners. They do so by attracting dust,
smoke, mold, pollen, bacteria, and viruses, all of which have a
positive charge. The heavier combined particle (the negative ion
plus the pollen, etc.) then falls from the air to the ground and is
removed from the breathing space. Negative ions have also been
shown to help reduce pain, heal burns, suppress mold and bacterial growth, stimulate plant growth, and contribute greatly to
our sense of well-being and comfort. Positive ions, on the other
hand, are air molecules lacking electrons. Pollen can carry fifty
or more positive charges per grain of pollen. This positive charge
slows the cilia and the clearing of mucus, and in so doing can
cause some degree of nasal congestion. Most man-made pollutants
result from combustion processes (auto/truck exhaust, smoke-
stacks, cigarette smoke, etc.) that leave the pollutants with a positive charge. Heating and ventilation systems tend to produce air
containing an excess of positive ions. Aircraft cabins have been
tested and found to contain an excessively high amount of positive ions. This obviously contributes to the "stuffy" feeling of
airplane air, and also helps to explain why so many of my patients have developed colds and sinus infections following air
travel. Television and especially computer screens also emit an
excess of positive ions, which draws negative ions out of the air

and neutralizes them. This may contribute (along with poor posture) to the frequent headaches experienced by people spending extended periods of time operating a computer.

The negative ion content of indoor air can be as low as 10 to 200 negative ions per cubic centimeter. This is considered to be "ion-depleted" air and is a significant component of "sick-building syndrome." Ion-depleted air is also created by heating/cooling systems, window air conditioners, and even air cleaners (including HEPA filters), which "scrub" negative ions from the air. Most of the factors in our environment responsible for depleting the beneficial negative ions also produce an excess of unhealthy positive ions.

The majority of Americans spend 90 percent of their time indoors, where, the EPA says, the air can be as much as 100 times more polluted than outdoor air. Few of us live in clean, moist environments that are warm year-round; even fewer live in the mountains, on a beach, or in the woods. For the 92 million people whose lungs, sinuses, and noses are already adversely affected from breathing unhealthy air, for the headache sufferer, and for anyone else who wants to enjoy optimum health, here are some ways to minimize the risks of breathing poor-quality air and to help prevent headache, asthma, sinusitis, and allergies.

HEALTHY HOMES

Where we live, work, play, or otherwise spend our time is critical to our health. If you are considering a move, you should look for a home in a location that minimizes the impact of outdoor air pollution or in a city or town that has minimal air pollution. If you are going to relocate and have the freedom to choose, avoid the following regions: southern California, the Northeast, and the Texas Gulf Coast. The healthiest air can be found along the West Coast (with the distinct exception of the Los Angeles metropolitan area and southward), rural areas along the Gulf Coast (other than Texas), and the west coast of Florida.

If you are contemplating the construction of a new home, the concept of *ecological architecture* could help considerably in creating a healthy environment. *Ecology* is defined in Webster's *New World Dictionary* as "the branch of biology that deals with the relationship between living organisms and their environment." Used as a modifier for the word *architecture,* it simply means the design of a dwelling that is sensitive to human health and gentle to the earth. Once we have considered the microclimate and the site, our biological needs, behavior patterns, and, most important, our budgetary limitations, nature will then dictate the design. Self-sufficiency through use of sun, air, earth, and water for heating, cooling, ventilation, and even electrical power is a realistic goal of an ecological design.

Common objectives regarding construction methods and materials include:

- avoiding the use of plastic or other materials made of toxic ingredients that harmfully outgas (give off toxins and/or fumes) in the indoor environment
- using nontoxic natural materials in preference to synthetic materials
- designing with concern for sensitivities, allergies, or chronic health problems
- being aware that nature's ecologic sustainability and well-being should not be diminished by what is built, and
- taking the responsibility to conceive, design, build, and furnish a home or building to a "healthy home" ecological ethic.

This is a holistic approach emphasizing the ecological bond between site and architecture. Preservation and wise use of our planet's resources in construction and throughout the lifetime of a home is fundamental to ecological design. For the headache, asthmatic, allergy, or sinus sufferer, a home must be clean, moist, warm, and oxygen- and negative ion–rich. The fact that it is designed in harmony with the atmosphere and the earth makes this an environmentally healthy concept.

I fully appreciate that most readers of this book will neither move nor design their own home as a result of what they read here. However, I want to present as many environmental treatment options as possible. Each can potentially benefit your headaches, and have a profound impact on your overall state of health and ultimately your quality of life. Fortunately, technology has made it possible to create an oasis of healthy indoor air in your own home, so you won't have to move or build a new home. In the desert an oasis provides water. In the sea of hazardous air in which we live, a *healthy home* or business can provide an oasis in which to breathe life-enhancing air.

Solving the problem of indoor air pollution entails both treatment and prevention. There is a company in Denver, Healthy Habitats, that has been on the leading edge of this field for more than twelve years. The owner of the company, Carl Grimes, has worked with me and a number of my patients to transform our unhealthy homes and offices into healthy ones. The procedures and techniques he employs adhere to the following guidelines:

- Prevention—avoid bringing pollutants into the home and workplace.
- Identify the source and develop a plan for isolating or removing the pollutant from the "breathing zone," or the surrounding area from which you obtain your breathing air, e.g., an infant's breathing zone includes the floor and carpeting.
- Reduce ambient pollution with ventilation, filtration, and ionization.

Grimes considers the three primary sources of pollution to be:

- Particulates—dust, pollen, dander, construction debris, and smoke
- Microorganisms—bacteria, viruses, molds, and dust mites
- Chemicals and gases—personal care products, cleaning products, office equipment, and building/construction materials (Refer to Table 4.1, pages 67 and 68.)

The type of treatment depends on the type of pollution. For example, HEPA filtration might be used for particulates, charcoal for chemicals and gases, and the drying of a wet crawl space could be the best option for eliminating microbes. Ozone has also been effective for persistent microorganisms; however, when a home is cleaned with ozone, the residents are advised to vacate the premises for two to three days. Chemical and gaseous pollution is harder to avoid than particulate matter and is probably a significant contributor to headaches. Although activated charcoal filters may be effective for removing toxic gases (formaldehyde is the most common gas found in homes), a simpler strategy involves the use of house plants known to absorb gases from the air (refer to page 77).

Table 4.1

Indoor Air Pollutants

Automotive Fumes
From outdoor traffic, outdoor parking lots, and outdoor loading and unloading spaces, as well as indoor garages

Chemicals and Chemical Solutions (Chemicals that affect indoor air quality are those associated with architecture, the interior, artifacts, and maintenance.)
Fungicides and pesticides in carpet-cleaning residues and sprays; formaldehyde, used in the manufacture of insulation, plywood, fiberboard, furniture, and wood paneling; toxic solvents in oil-based paints, finishes, and wall sealants; aerosol sprays; office equipment chemicals, especially photocopiers and computers

Combustion Products
Tobacco smoke★
Coal- or wood-burning fireplaces and stoves
Fuel combustion gases from gas-fired appliances such as ranges, clothes dryers, water heaters, and fireplaces (they produce nitro-

gen dioxide, carbon monoxide, nitrous oxides, sulfur oxides, hydrocarbons, and formaldehyde)

Ion Depletion or Imbalance
Too few negative ions
Excess of positive ions over negative ions

Microorganisms (primarily from humidifiers, air conditioners, and any other building components affected by excessive moisture)
Bacteria
Viruses
Molds
Dust mites (usually found in more humid areas)

Particulates
Dust
Pollen
Animal dander
Particles (frayed materials)
Asbestos

Radionuclides
Radon, a radioactive gas emitted from the earth that enters homes primarily through basements, crawl spaces, and water supply, especially from wells (it can attach to the particulates of cigarette smoke, dust particles, and natural aerosols)

*From all of the available scientific data, tobacco smoke is the most unhealthy indoor air pollutant.

Molds are rapidly becoming one of America's chief health hazards and are recognized as one of the leading causes for the dramatic increase in asthma, allergies, and chronic sinusitis during the past twenty years. Although it is not definitively known, molds are probably also a significant headache trigger. The reason many of us are being exposed daily to high levels of mold is primarily a result of modern home design—more airtight, with air-conditioning and heating systems recirculating contaminated air; materials used; and most important, *water leaks.* Molds can grow wherever it's damp, so it's important to quickly fix any leaks, regularly clean air ducts and furnace filters, be on the lookout for discoloration of walls or ceilings and any unusual odors, and empty (daily) and clean (weekly) humidifiers on a regular basis.

Several excellent books are available on the subject of healthy homes. Those that I recommend are: *Starting Points for a Healthy Habitat* by Carl Grimes (Healthy Habitats); *The Nontoxic Home and Office* by Debra Lynn Dadd (Jeremy P. Tarcher, Inc.); *The Healthy House* by John Bower (Lyle Stuart, Inc.); and *Your Home, Your Health and Well-Being* by David Rousseau (Ten Speed Press).

Air Cleaners and Negative-Ion Generators

As many as one million hospital admissions a year are attributed to poor indoor air quality. In recent years, as the EPA and private health organizations have publicized the problem of indoor air pollution, we have seen a proliferation of several hundred types of air cleaners, almost as many as there are indoor air pollutants. According to Michael Berry, Ph.D., former manager of

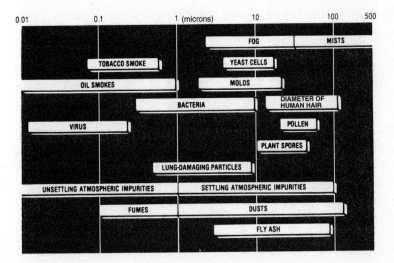

FIGURE 4.1. *Relative size of common air contaminants.*

the EPA's Indoor Air Project, the most potentially harmful pollutants are radon and the "biologicals," including pollen, molds, plant spores, dust mites, bacteria, and viruses. The pollutants most harmful to the respiratory tract are less than one micron in size. Regardless of their origin, size, or health-damaging effects, air pollutants can be described as free-floating particles in the air. Figure 4.1 shows the specific size ranges of the most common pollutants. The unit of measurement used for tiny air particles is the micron. An average hair strand is 100 microns thick, and about 400 one-micron particles would fit into the dot over the *i* in the word *micron*. The primary job of air cleaners is to remove as many of these particles as possible, the biologicals as well as the combustion products, particulates, chemicals, fumes, and odors. (See Figure 4.1, page 69.) Radon, if present, requires the sealing of basement cracks and improvement of basement ventilation. Most air cleaners do not remove radon from the air. However, some air cleaners with high particle removal efficiency (HEPA, etc.) can remove some of the radon "daughters" (attached radon) that are in particulate form. A study at the Harvard School of Public Health determined that a negative-ion generator is a highly effective means of removing the attached fraction of radon (the radon daughters), although it does not reduce the unattached (gaseous) fraction of radon.

The strategy for solving the problem of indoor air pollution involves *air cleaning* and *improved ventilation*. Air-cleaning devices can include furnace filters, portable stand-alone units, and negative-ion generators. The efficiency of air cleaners is evaluated by their ability to filter a certain percentage of a certain size of pollutant. The HEPA filter (an acronym for high-efficiency particulate arrestor) removes 97 percent of all 0.3-micron particulates and larger. This includes pollen, mold, plant spores, most animal dander, dust, wood, and tobacco smoke, fumes, bacteria, and some viruses. This type of filter is standard equipment for most hospital operating suites, and is found in many of the more expensive freestanding air cleaners. It requires a strong fan or a booster fan to move air through it due to its increased efficiency.

The ULPA (Ultra Low Penetrating Air) filters were originally created to purify the air in semiconductor clean rooms. The Bionaire company has now made this new technology available to clean the air in homes. ULPA air purifiers are equipped with a superfine filter that removes a remarkable 99.999 percent of all airborne particles as small as 0.1 micron. The filter traps such allergens as tobacco smoke, pollen, dust, dust mites, mold, and bacteria. For best performance, it is recommended that ULPA filters be changed every six months to one year.

Negative-ion generators were originally designed to restore a more natural and beneficial level of negative ions to indoor air. In the course of their use for biological benefit, it was discovered that free-floating ions quickly attach to airborne particles and cause them to agglomerate and precipitate from the air, or be drawn to grounded surfaces such as walls, metal surfaces, and so on. Ionizers are highly effective air cleaners, removing particles as small as .001 micron, which would include viruses, molds, dust, pollen, cigarette smoke, and all other airborne particulate pollutants. Compared to air cleaners with fans or blowers, ionizers are more likely to be operated full-time since they are totally silent (no fan) and consume only pennies of electricity per month.

However, in order to increase the speed with which an ionizer cleans the air, many manufacturers produce ionizers with excessive ion output. This has two undesirable effects: (1) The ion density established by these ionizers exceeds many times the natural range found outdoors, resulting in much the same adverse effects as breathing air with too few negative ions. A well-designed negative-ion generator will generate enough ions to be effective but will not exceed an upper limit that would make it biologically undesirable. (2) An excessively high ion density also causes a significant amount of pollutants to be driven to the walls and other grounded surfaces, resulting in the buildup of a dirty residue. Again, a well-designed ion generator will minimize such "plating," and this effect can be further reduced by placing the ionizer at least two feet from the nearest wall.

It has been my good fortune, and that of my patients, to have worked with a "pioneer" in negative-ion technology. For nearly thirty years Rex Coppom, owner of Electrofilter Technologies in Longmont, Colorado, has been developing state-of-the-art negative-ion generators. For almost ten years many of my patients have been using his Sinus Survival Air Vitalizer, a small unit that will clean the air of a 150- to 200-square-foot room. Its self-regulation feature enables it to maintain an ideal level of negative ions (3,000 to 6,000 per cubic centimeter). It costs $150, considerably less than the average price of a HEPA room air cleaner, which is somewhat less efficient in its cleaning capacity and has no negative ions. I have received many testimonials about its beneficial effects—dramatic headache relief, fewer allergy and asthma attacks, diminished nasal congestion, cessation of snoring, better sleep, more energy, general feelings of well-being, and diminished odor and symptoms resulting from secondhand cigarette smoke. I was amazed at how quickly it cleared the smoke from my kitchen during an oven-cleaning session that went somewhat awry. Ionization equipment is currently available for automobiles and aircraft cabins—both of which have far less than optimum air.

Electronic air cleaners (both central and freestanding) produce positive ions as they filter the air. On their first day of operation they are 85 percent efficient on all 1-micron particles and larger, but in order to maintain that efficiency they require cleaning every two weeks. For most of us, this makes them impractical and inconvenient. They also produce ozone, which can be a potential health hazard.

To obtain a *furnace filter,* go to a hardware or building-supply store. Many of them carry the 3M pleated filter, under the brand name Filtret. These are excellent furnace filters and cost about $15. They should be replaced every one to two months during the winter and while central air conditioners are being run regularly. They are far more efficient than the $2 to $4 varieties found in supermarkets. There are several other brands of pleated furnace filters that are similar in efficiency to 3M.

The Dupont Wizard dustcloth is an interesting product that does a better job of dusting than can be obtained from liquid or spray dust cleaners. They are used dry, can be washed, and cost $2.

Air Duct Cleaning

When the air duct system of my thirteen-year-old home was cleaned for the first time, I was amazed at what emanated from the ducts after two hours of high-intensity vacuuming. I thought to myself, "It's no wonder I suffered with sinus problems for so long!" If the air ducts are filthy, it is nearly impossible for your furnace filter to clean the air in your home. After the air is filtered, it still has to travel through the ducts before you breathe it. I recommend air duct cleaning as part of the environmental treatment program. Depending on the size of your home, an air duct cleaning service, using good equipment, could cost between $200 and $250. To find this type of company in your city, look in the Yellow Pages under "Furnaces, Cleaning and Repairing."

Carpet Cleaning

Carpets are one of the most common sources of indoor air pollutants. They are excellent traps and hold on to dust, pollen, and microorganisms. While this helps to keep those particles out of the breathing zone, their gradual accumulation can become great enough to create a sustainable culture of bacteria, yeast, dust mites, and mold. In fact, many allergists recommend that their patients dispose of all their carpets.

While it is true that carpets harbor pollutants, it is possible to keep them clean. This poses a challenge to the homemaker. Conventional vacuum cleaners are designed to remove and retain the visible dirt, which means particles greater than 10 microns. Most of the particles and microorganisms that are too small to be seen are also smaller than the pores in the vacuum cleaner bag. This allows most of them to blow through the bag and into the room, settling back onto the carpets and furniture.

If a forced-air heating system is running, the airborne particles can be drawn into the air ducts, contributing to their contamination as well. Also, as the bag fills, airflow decreases, causing uneven cleaning.

To prevent these problems I suggest a vacuum cleaner that uses either a HEPA-type filter or water capture. Either one can remove subvisible dust and bacteria from the air. The water-capture types also have a continuously maximum airflow because they won't clog like a bag or filter. Both of these vacuums are expensive, costing between $500 and $1,000.

However, there is a much less expensive alternative. Dupont Hysurf vacuum cleaner bags have 1-micron pores and cost only $5. They appear to have the equivalent cleaning efficiency of the $500-plus "allergy" vacuum cleaners. Their major problem is that they are difficult to find. Some janitorial supply houses and medical supply stores have them. They can also be obtained from Thriving Health Products.

Many people have their carpets professionally cleaned. However, due to their chemical composition, the most common cleaning agents are often worse than having dirty carpets. Alcohols, petroleum distillates, ammonia, dry-cleaning substances, and scents often cause headaches, mental "fuzziness," lethargy, and a general feeling of discomfort. Cleaning-agent residues may often cause respiratory irritation.

Before contracting with a carpet cleaner, check his references and insist on a nonscented cleaning agent that uses no petroleum distillates, alcohol, ammonia, dry-cleaning-type chemicals or enzymes, and has no suds that can be left in the carpet. Check his work to be sure he leaves no damp areas. This ensures maximum removal of all agents and enhances drying time. If the carpet stays wet for several days, bacteria and molds can grow rapidly.

Ventilation and Plants

All indoor spaces, whether residential, commercial, industrial, or recreational, require some type of ventilation to provide breathable air for occupants, to furnish combustion air for cooking and heating, and to remove stale air filled with toxins and particulates. Commercial buildings are required by code to have even more efficient ventilation systems than residences. The American Society of Heating, Refrigerating and Air-Conditioning Engineers (ASHRAE) says that air should be replaced at the rate of 15 cubic feet per minute per person, but most systems fall below this minimum standard.

Improving ventilation will help relieve indoor air pollution as long as the outdoor air isn't dirtier than the air it is replacing. Local pollution sources, such as fumes from toxic waste leakage, wood burning, a neighboring industrial plant, a heavily trafficked highway, or crop spraying can render outdoor air unacceptable for indoor ventilation. Several days a year Los Angeles residents are advised to keep all windows and doors closed and ventilation ducts shut to prevent the heavily polluted outdoor air from entering homes and businesses. In areas like this it becomes a challenge to balance the health benefit of highly oxygenated outdoor air and the liability of the pollutants that come with it. Outdoor aerobic exercise presents a similar dilemma. If you live in a heavily polluted environment, I recommend exercising outside and ventilating your home and office well when outdoor air is good, but exercise indoors and keep windows and doors closed during periods of heavy pollution.

Air-conditioning systems are a helpful means of ventilation for people with headaches triggered by air pollution, asthma, and allergy problems. These systems remove excess moisture from the air, lowering its temperature. In less humid conditions there is a reduction of molds and spores, and with the windows closed there is also a marked decrease in pollutants and pollen from the outdoors. Air-conditioning, however, does deplete negative ions from the air.

Natural cross-ventilation is effective in reducing indoor air pollution if the placement of the intake vents is low and the outlets for the flow-through air are high. Operable windows on commercial buildings and a good location for the outdoor air intake—away from garage entrances or loading docks—are also important factors in improving indoor air quality. Mechanical ventilation with exhaust fans can certainly help in removing indoor pollutants, but such fans are most efficient when used in a confined space. Private offices or single-occupant rooms where smoking, cooking, and other fume-producing activities take place are ideal environments for mechanical ventilation.

Rooms producing commercial toxic or odoriferous fumes; spaces subject to bacterial and viral contamination, such as rest rooms; and indoor areas that present specific respiratory hazards all need optimized ventilation. Mold is a special problem in moist conditions. Adequate ventilation along with sunshine can help to reduce moisture and subsequently suppress mold.

The technology of ventilation can be complex, but the basic principle of displacing interior air with outdoor air and increasing the rate of fresh airflow is critical to treating the problem of indoor air pollution. Besides natural cross-ventilation and exhaust fans, other devices used to enhance ventilation and indoor air quality are air-to-air heat exchangers, makeup air units, attic fans, vortex fans, and ceiling fans. Remember that even if the "fresh" air is filthy, an effective air cleaner combined with good ventilation is still a winning combination.

Adequate ventilation not only helps reduce indoor air pollution but is the primary source of indoor oxygen. Plants can offer an aesthetically pleasant secondary source in addition to their ability to remove toxic gases from the air. *Plants can help improve indoor air as oxygenators, filters, and humidifiers.* Although the oxygen output from indoor plants is not great, plants with large leaf surfaces that grow rapidly are capable of enhancing air quality. Attached greenhouses and atria filled with plants that effectively absorb carbon dioxide and oxygenate the air (spider plants do this very well) can improve the indoor environment while humidifying the air.

In the early 1990s, studies conducted at the John Stennis Space Center in Mississippi showed that plants can also act as effective filters. Former NASA scientist Bill C. Wolverton, Ph.D., has spent the past thirty years studying the ability of plants to clear volatile organic chemicals from indoor air. Wolverton predicts that within twenty years plants will be governmentally mandated in new buildings as a matter of public health.

According to the EPA, the most plentiful of the organic chemicals in the average indoor environment is formaldehyde. It is released from a host of household furnishings, including synthetic carpeting, particleboard (used to make bookcases, desks, and tables), foam insulation, upholstery, curtains, and even so-called air fresheners. Common house plants such as chrysanthemums, striped dracaena, dwarf date palms, and especially Boston ferns are excellent filters for removing formaldehyde. Spider plants are also effective in removing carbon monoxide; areca palms are best at filtering xylene, the second-most-prevalent indoor organic chemical; and English ivy is good for filtering benzene, ranked third on the EPA's list. Aloe vera, philodendron, pothos, and ficus were also found to reduce levels of organic chemicals.

The Foliage for Clean Air Council, a communications clearinghouse for information on the use of foliage to improve indoor air quality, recommends a minimum of two plants per 100 square feet of floor space in an average home with eight- to ten-foot ceilings.

Prevention

Prevention of indoor air pollution involves eliminating pollutants at the source. Doctors who specialize in environmental medicine and some allergists can do skin and blood tests to help you identify pollutants to which you are particularly sensitive (headache triggers) or allergic. These doctors are not always easy to find, nor are the tests always definitive, but they can help. With the use of environmentally sensitive architectural principles, a healthier home can be created. A major preventive strategy is the use of interior materials that emit no pollutants. Natural products such as wood, cotton, and metals are preferable to the lower-cost synthetic materials such as particleboard, fiberboard, polyester, and plastics.

Choosing to forgo a fireplace or wood-burning stove would be helpful, as would using a high-efficiency furnace with a sealed combustion unit to vent exhaust gases to the outside. Switch to nontoxic cleaning substances, including ordinary soap, vinegar, zephiran, and Air Therapy. (You can find a listing of such cleaners in *Nontoxic, Natural, & Earthwise,* by Debra Lynn Dadd.) Smoking should be relegated to the outdoors or to a well-ventilated enclosed space. If radon levels exceed the acceptable EPA standard of 4 picoCuries per liter of air, radon control measures should be implemented. Formaldehyde from insulation can be eliminated by using the substitutes of cellulose and white fiberglass insulation.

BREATHING

Oxygen is the most critical nutrient for every cell in the body. It is literally the "spark of life" needed to provide energy for every basic bodily function. Breathing is our constant and immediate connection to life: we can go days without water, weeks without food, but only minutes without oxygen. *Headache is usually the first physical sign of a lack of oxygen.* We begin life with our first breath, and end it with our last. During our adult life we normally breathe about 23,000 times a day without ever giving much thought to this miraculous process. Because respiration, synchronized with heartbeat, is an automatic function, we are seldom aware of how we breathe, or attempt to breathe more efficiently or healthfully, until we are confronted with the crisis of having great difficulty breathing—for example, an asthma attack, being in a smoke-filled room, or being at high altitude. These frightening, often terrifying situations instantaneously alert us to the vital need for oxygen. Suddenly you become intimately aware of your own breath, your heart rate, muscle tension, your anxiety and fear. Your breath is labored and you feel yourself fighting to breathe to save your life. The harder you struggle to breathe, the more rapid and shallow your breaths become, decreasing the available amount of oxygen. According to recent research, over-breathing, or hyperventilation, might be a primary factor in triggering an asthmatic attack. It is now known that *hyperventilation is also a common cause of headaches.* Medical professor Konstantin Buteyko, a Russian researcher, has performed extensive experiments in Russia for more than forty-five years on the effects of overbreathing. This led him to the controversial theory that hyperventilation is a primary *cause* of ailments such as asthma and headaches. He defines hyperventilation as the habitual inhalation of more than 4 to 6 liters of air per minute—considered to be the normal rate of respiration. It is the equivalent of 8 to 12 breaths per minute, with each breath being the equivalent of a pint of air, or about two gallons per minute. In contrast, a person practiced in slow, rhythmic breathing may inhale 5 liters over a 3-minute period, or a rate between 3 and 4 breaths per minute. With hyperventilation secondary to stress (a headache trigger), it can be as high as 10 to 15 liters during a 1-minute period—as much as 20 to 30 breaths per minute. In addition to the lack of oxygen, this type of breathing also lowers carbon dioxide excessively.

Professor Buteyko recognized carbon dioxide as not just a waste product, but an important chemical regulator that is essential for the *utilization* of oxygen in the cells. Chronic overbreathing creates a deficiency of carbon dioxide, which increases potential for muscle spasm and decreases *available* oxygen. By teaching patients techniques of slow, periodic underbreathing he found that he could effect a significant reduction in asthma symptoms in 90 percent of his patients. Teresa Hale, founder of the highly regarded Hale Clinic in London (the United Kingdom's largest holistic medical clinic with over one hundred practitioners, including thirty M.D.s), has confirmed Buteyko's findings and claims his breathing techniques have produced dramatic reductions in asthma symptoms in just five days. She, too, found that it worked for 90 percent of their patients. She has proven similar success with applying the technique to headache sufferers. To date, over one million people in the former Soviet Union have applied this technique with similar results. (For more in-depth information about Buteyko's Method, refer to the book *Breathing Free* by Teresa Hale, listed in the bibliography.)

These breathing techniques can be used for countering hyperventilation or in any situation where there is a lack of oxygen. Today, a growing number of researchers and practitioners are concluding that breathing techniques that emphasize the out breath, while breathing slowly and through the nose, are highly effective. Regardless of the cause, the lack of oxygen can provide you with an opportunity to learn how to intervene and consciously take control of breathing effectively. Obviously, learning to breathe more efficiently and taking in more oxygen is also a key component to reducing headache and experiencing optimal health. You can choose to see your headaches from hyperventilation, usually caused by anxiety and stress, as warnings your body is sending you, and use the experience as an opportunity to begin practicing more conscious and effective breathing—an act of loving your body. Breathing this way can help to break the cycle of anxiety and shortness of breath that accompany muscle tension and pain. As your lungs become better conditioned, it becomes easier to practice. Conscious breathing allows you to be much more in control and no longer a victim.

By learning to be more aware of your breathing patterns and applying a time-honored blend of traditional yogic techniques with newer, clinically proven methods, you will be able to lessen the frequency, duration, and intensity of headaches resulting from hyperventilation. Since stress is most often the trigger for hyperventilation, this type of breathing will help you to reduce stress and learn to relax.

In this chapter I will coach you on a beginning level of breathing exercises. At the end of this section I will direct you to resources for more advanced techniques. Consider this as the first step in putting your lungs into "breathing training camp" in order to condition them for consistently better function. You do not need to have headaches to benefit from these breathing techniques. The exercises help to strengthen peripheral and accessory breathing muscles that assist the lungs, thereby relieving the workload of the diaphragm. Most of us have an estimated 20 percent of unused lung capacity at any given time. When your lungs are trained to do so, you can draw on this reserve during times of respiratory distress.

Most people with headaches have a heightened state of chronic muscle tension combined with exhaustion. This is because there is a long-term imbalance in the sympathetic and parasympathetic branches of the nervous system. The parasympathetic branch is like a "brake," creating relaxation, full and easy breathing, sleep, and good digestion. The sympathetic branch acts as the "accelerator." It rouses us to action and puts us into the "fight-or-flight" stress response when we perceive a threat. During the fight-or-flight response, adrenaline is released and breathing becomes shallow and rapid, heart rate and blood pressure go up, and muscles become tense in preparation for action. Many headache sufferers live highly stressed lives resulting in a condition of fight-or-flight breathing—a state of stressful, excessive sympathetic nervous function, which can potentially exhaust the lungs and the adrenal glands. This state of sympathetic excess causes a form of chronic hyperventilation, or overbreathing, and leads to a constant state of hypoxia, or low oxygen in the bloodstream. Hypoxia, in turn, can heighten anxiety and fatigue, which can significantly increase the frequency and intensity of headaches.

The Headache Survival approach to effective breathing techniques synthesizes the principles I have just discussed and starts you on five of the most important exercises. Remember to begin slowly, listen to your body's feedback, and practice at least once or twice a day for 5 minutes each time. (Many people choose to practice for a few minutes every hour. This is even more effective.) If for any reason you feel light-headed or out of breath, just take a minute or two to breathe normally and relax. Then try resuming the exercise again. If your sinuses are congested, then I recommend that you steam and do nasal irrigation prior to the exercises to open the nasal passages. If at all possible, try to perform these exercises in a clean air environment.

1. Basic Belly (or abdominal) Breathing
Begin by lying on your back with your knees up and legs slightly apart. Get comfortable and at first just notice your breathing without trying to do anything. Relax and feel yourself

"sinking" into the floor. Then place your open hands around your lower rib cage, with your palms at the lower part of your ribs and your fingertips touching at your belly button. Feel the lower parts of your ribs expand and your belly rise up easily and smoothly as you breathe in through your nose. Now breathe out long and slow through your nose or mouth as you feel your belly sink. When breathing out through your mouth keep your lips close together, firmly pushing the air out. Try not to engage your shoulders or upper chest in the breathing effort. See if you can comfortably breath out for 4 to 5 seconds or more and in for 1 to 3 seconds. Go slowly, don't overbreathe, let the breath out long and slow while you relax and sink deeper into the floor. The out breath will relax you more and more. Breathing out

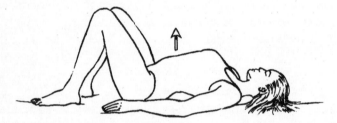

FIGURE 4.2

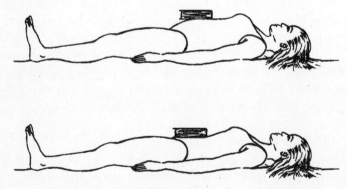

FIGURE 4.3

will create air hunger and naturally encourage an inhalation. Let the in breath be slow, smooth, and through the nose. Feel the inhale deep in the back of your throat, but *do not take in a forced, large inhalation.* Remember that you want to emphasize a complete out breath. Try working toward breathing out for 8 to 12 seconds and in for 2 to 4. To feel your belly muscles even more, you may want to place a book or something that has some added weight on your abdomen for kinesthetic feedback. Once you are comfortable with this exercise, add a variation; at the end of the outbreath, try to hum, or add an MMMM or NNNNN sound to expel even more residual air.

2. Belly Breathing while seated

Use the same instructions as above, but while sitting in a chair. Keep your hands wrapped around your lower ribs to get a good feel of the muscular action. This is good to do at the office, in class, even in traffic—but keep both hands on the wheel!

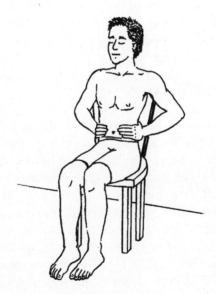

FIGURE 4.4

3. Belly Breathing while walking
Try walking for 5 to 15 minutes at a time, once daily. Start slowly and remember to focus on the out breath, starting with a count of 4 out and 2 in. Try adding 2 counts on the out breath over time but keeping the in breath shorter. The basic rule is that the exhalation should be at least two times longer than the inhalation. Over a period of weeks or months, depending on your condition, try building the count on the out breath to more than 10. Try adding a light hissing or whooshing sound from your lips while exhaling once you are tolerating the exercise well. Be patient and persistent. This helps condition the lungs for longer endurance and aerobic conditioning. Once you are tolerating this exercise well, you may want to try it on a mini-trampoline, also called a rebounder, while gently bouncing. The bouncing motion promotes lymphatic circulation and oxygenation.

Conditioned belly breathing can significantly help to reduce the intensity, duration, and frequency of your headaches (especially tension). At the same time you will learn an effective method of relaxation while expanding your capacity to thrive, with much more energy and vitality and a greater sense of aliveness.

2. Water and Moisture

Next to oxygen, *water*, the second of the essential 8 for optimal health, is our most important nutrient, and drinking enough water to satisfy your body's needs may be the simplest, least expensive (other than belly/abdominal breathing) self-help measure you can adopt to maintain your overall good health. Sufficient water can also help to prevent headaches resulting from the inflamed mucous membranes, thick mucus, and congestion of chronic sinusitis or from dehydration. It has been estimated that a 1 percent dehydration in the muscle can lead to an 8–10 percent energy loss in the muscles, thereby increasing potential for spasm, pain, and tension.

Our adult bodies are 60 to 70 percent water (an infant's body is about 80 percent), and water is the medium through which every bodily function occurs. It is the basis of all body fluids, including blood, digestive juices, urine, lymph, and perspiration, which explains why we would die within a few days without water.

Water is vital to metabolism and digestion and helps prevent both constipation and diarrhea. It is also critical to healthy nerve impulse conduction and brain function. Some of water's other vital functions in the body are:

- Enhancing oxygen uptake into the bloodstream (the surface of the lungs must be moistened with water to facilitate oxygen intake and the excretion of carbon dioxide)
- Maintaining a high urine volume, helping to prevent kidney stones and urinary tract infections
- Regulating body temperature through perspiration
- Maintaining and increasing the health of the skin
- Maintaining adequate fluid for the lubrication of the joints and enhancing muscular function, particularly during and after exercise or other strenuous activity
- Moistening the mucous membranes of the respiratory tract, which in turn increases resistance to infection and thins the mucus, allowing it to drain more easily

Because water is so important to our health, all of us need to make a conscious effort to stay well hydrated, since most of us lose water faster than we replace it. For example, we lose one pint of water each day simply through exhalation. We also lose the same amount through perspiration, as well as three additional pints per day through urination and defecation. Exercise and heat exposure, especially in a dry climate, also increase water loss in the body. The percentage of body water content also decreases with age. All told, on average, each of us loses two and a half quarts of water (80 ounces) per day under normal conditions. Therefore, it is essential that the same amount or more be replenished daily.

Unfortunately, most Americans don't come close to consuming that much water per day. As a result, many of us are chronically dehydrated. When we think of dehydration, we may envision a lost soul in the desert, dying of thirst. However, most conditions of dehydration are not that dramatic, so that dehydration all too often is unsuspected and therefore undiagnosed. Meanwhile, its insidious effects can wreak havoc on our health by chronically impacting every one of our bodily functions. The results are:

- Reduced blood volume, with less oxygen and nutrients provided to all muscles and organs (*headaches can result from even mild dehydration,* causing less oxygen to be provided to the brain)
- Reduced brain size and impaired neuromuscular coordination, concentration, and thinking
- Excess body fat
- Poor muscle tone and size
- Impaired digestive function and constipation
- Increased toxicity in the body
- Joint and muscle pain
- Water retention (edema), which can result in a state of being overweight and also impede weight loss
- Hyperconcentration of blood with increased viscosity, leading to higher risk of heart attack.

Even though you may not be feeling thirsty, you may nonetheless be one of the millions of Americans who are chronically dehydrated. Observation of your urine is one simple way to determine if you are. If your urine is heavy, cloudy, and deep yellow, orange, or brown in tint, it's more than likely that you are dehydrated. The urine of a properly hydrated body tends to be light and nearly clear in color, similar in appearance to unsweetened lemonade. As your water intake approaches your daily need for it, you will notice the appearance of your urine changing accordingly. (Remember that B vitamins will also turn urine a dark yellow.)

Because dehydration is so deceptive—it can occur without

symptoms of thirst—in general, we need to drink more water than our thirst calls for. This does not mean coffee, soft drinks, or alcohol, all of which contribute further to dehydration. Even processed fruit juices and milk are not healthy substitutes for water, because of the sugar and possible pesticides in the former and the hormones and antibiotics in the latter.

The exact amount of water a person needs depends on a number of individual factors, such as body weight, diet, metabolic rate, climate, level of physical activity, and stress factors. Some health professionals recommend that we all drink 8 eight-ounce glasses of water a day. A more accurate rule of thumb is to drink half an ounce of water per pound of body weight if you are a healthy but sedentary adult, and to increase that amount to two-thirds of an ounce per pound if you are an active exerciser. This means that a healthy, sedentary adult weighing 160 pounds should drink about 10 eight-ounce glasses of water per day, while an active exerciser should drink 13 to 14 eight-ounce glasses. If your diet is particularly high in fresh fruits and vegetables, your daily water intake needs may be less, since these foods are 85 to 90 percent water in content and can help restore lost fluids. Herbal teas, natural fruit juices (without sugar added and diluted 50 percent with water), and soups that are sugarless and low in salt (the thinner the better) are also acceptable substitutes for drinking water.

Nearly as important as the amount of water you drink is the *quality* of your water. Simply put, if you aren't drinking filtered water, then your body is forced to become the filter. Still, it's impossible to generalize about whether you should drink tap, bottled, or filtered water. (Distilled water is not recommended for drinking because it lacks necessary minerals and can also leach them from your body.) In some communities, water purity is so high that it requires no treatment, while other water sources are contaminated with high concentrations of lead and radon, the two worst contaminants.

Another issue related to our drinking water is chlorination. Since chlorine was first introduced into America's drinking water supply in 1908, it has eliminated epidemics of cholera, dysentery, and typhoid. Multiple studies, however, now suggest an association between chlorine and increased free radical production, which can lead to a higher incidence of cancer. On the positive side, chlorine is effective in eliminating most microorganisms from drinking water. (One notable exception is the parasite *Cryptosporidium,* which is resistant to chlorine.)

Unless you live in one of the communities that supply pure water, drinking tap water is not recommended, especially since the majority of health-related risks present in drinking water occur from contamination that is added *after* the water leaves the treatment and distribution plant. This includes pipes that run from municipal systems into your home, lead-soldered copper pipes, and fixtures that contain lead and may leach lead or other toxic metals (such as cadmium, mercury, and cobalt) into your tap water. Therefore, if you drink tap water, it would be a good idea to have the water from your tap tested, regardless of the claims from your local water utility. You can get started by calling your local health department for a referral for testing.

Because of the growing concerns regarding tap water, increasing numbers of Americans now choose bottled water for drinking and cooking purposes. This can not only prove to be expensive, but also may not be as safe as you think. Regulations mandated for the bottled-water industry are similar to those followed by the public water treatment industry and currently do not include required testing for *Cryptosporidium* and many other contaminants. Moreover, 25 percent of bottled water sold in this country comes from filtered municipal water that is then treated. For this reason, perhaps the healthiest choice regarding your drinking water is to invest in a water filter. Reverse-osmosis filters appear to be the most effective home water-filtering systems presently available. But there are also some distillation and carbon filters that are able to reduce lead in water significantly. There are carafe-style filters for the kitchen faucet that cost about $25, under-the-sink models for $400, and point-of-entry units that purify the water as it enters the house. These can cost as much as $1,250.

Since it is impossible to always know for certain whether

what we drink or eat is completely safe, do the best you can. To get in the habit of drinking enough water, spread your intake throughout the day (drinking very little after dinner), and don't drink more than four eight-ounce glasses in any one-hour period. It's also best to drink between meals so as not to interfere with your body's digestive process. Make your water drinking convenient; keep a container of water at hand, in your car, or at your desk, and don't wait until you feel thirsty to start drinking. Most important, be sure that there's always a bathroom nearby. The belief that you can stretch your bladder is a myth.

Humidification

In addition to drinking water, it is important to breathe moist air. From my clinical experience, having practiced in Denver for thirty years, it is obvious that extremely dry air can be irritating to the mucous membranes and can trigger sinus headaches. It can also be a significant contributing factor in sinus infections and asthmatic attacks, especially cold and dry air. According to Dr. Marshall Plaut, chief of the asthma and allergy branch at the National Institute of Allergy and Infectious Diseases (part of NIH), "Dry air triggers asthma and nasal congestion." Studies on patients with allergic rhinitis have shown that warm, moist air can improve nasal congestion and other allergy symptoms. Optimum indoor air quality requires air containing between 35 and 55 percent relative humidity. Moisture provided by room humidifiers can greatly benefit anyone with a respiratory condition and headaches secondary to irritated and/or inflamed sinuses. These humidifiers are most helpful in the winter, even in humid, cold-weather climates, because most heating systems dry the indoor air considerably. However, if you are sensitive to mold and believe that exposure to mold is a primary trigger of your headaches, then I would be more cautious about using a humidifier. Room humidifiers, also called tabletop models, have sufficient capacity to humidify a medium- to large-size room. Each type has some drawbacks. Ultrasonic models can emit an irritating white dust. So can cool-mist models, which require the use of distilled water or an expensive demineralization cartridge, unless you have very soft water. Steam-mist models, also called vaporizers, can scald if you get too close to the mist they produce or if you tip them over by accident. Evaporative models, the most prevalent type, can become a breeding ground for bacteria. The warm-mist units are my first choice. They produce a mist just slightly warmer than room air, use tap water, require no filter, and are able to kill bacteria. Their only drawback may be that they use more electricity than the other types. Most humidifiers are quiet and very effective in producing a moist environment in an enclosed space. They are available in pharmacies, department stores, and hardware stores under a variety of brand names. The one I know best and with which I have enjoyed excellent results is the Bionaire-Clear Mist 5 (CMP-5). It quietly yet powerfully puts out warm moisture, can cover an area of up to 1,600 square feet, and is relatively easy to clean. The Kenmore Warm Mist is the identical unit, and it is available at most Sears stores. These units cost about $125. Although the ideal humidifier has probably not yet been designed, I've recently tried the Slant/Fin GF-200. This warm mist humidifier uses ultraviolet germicidal technology to produce 99.999 percent germ-free mist. It costs under $100. The tabletop humidifiers can cost from $30 to $125.

The larger humidifiers, called consoles, can humidify an average-size house, cost from $100 to $200, and are all the evaporative type. Although I've had no personal experience with these, I know that *Consumer Reports* has given a high rating to the Bionaire W-6S, as well as to the Toastmaster 3435 and Emerson HD850.

Central or in-duct humidifiers, those that attach to the furnace, are more convenient but often do not humidify an individual room as well as a portable humidifier can when the door to the room is closed. In the past the major problem with central humidifiers has been that most of them were the reservoir type, with a tray of standing water that breeds mold and bacteria. I recommend the flow-through type of central humidifier—

for example, Aprilaire or General, which eliminates the stagnant water problem and is easy to maintain. Depending on the model, size of your home, and installation, this humidifier would probably cost about $250 to $650.

Humidifiers are not the only option for moisturizing your home. The installation of waterfalls, indoor spas, and swimming pools will all add a lot of moisture to the house, but of course they are expensive to install and maintain. It may surprise you to learn that even the moisture from human breath and sweat, along with that from cooking, baths, showers, and plants, adds significantly to a home's humidity. If your bedroom is dry, hang a wet towel on a hanger in the room.

If you rarely suffer jolts of static electricity when you touch metal objects such as doorknobs, then the air in your home is probably humid enough. For a more precise test, you'll need a hygrometer. You can find these humidity-measuring devices at most hardware stores. The one I've been using is the Bionaire Climate Check, a digital device that measures both temperature and humidity.

Another device I've been using preventively on myself and recommending to patients is the *steam inhaler*. It can be quite soothing to dry and irritated mucous membranes while also relieving sinus headaches. There is evidence that steam also helps to open your airway and can act as a decongestant and bronchodilator. A few drops or a spray of medicinal eucalyptus oil added to the unit while you are steaming enhances its therapeutic effect. For quick relief of a sinus headache I often recommend spraying this eucalyptus (Sinus Survival Eucalyptus Oil) on a tissue held close to the nose while inhaling it through the nose. To benefit the entire mucous membrane while steaming, alternate inhaling through your nose (upper respiratory tract) and your mouth (lower respiratory tract—lungs). If used just prior to nasal irrigation, it will greatly increase the benefit of the irrigation. The steam inhaler I use is made by Kaz and costs about $50, but unfortunately is no longer readily available. Information on where to obtain any of the products I mention is listed in the product index at the end of the book. For additional information on treating chronic sinusitis, please refer to the fourth edition of *Sinus Survival.*'

Assuming your environment is relatively dry, as indoor air tends to be during the winter months in most parts of the United States, you can also provide moisture with a *saltwater* (also called *saline*) *nasal spray.* There are several commercial products available in pharmacies. However, you can make your own saline spray by mixing one half of a teaspoon of non-iodized table salt and a pinch of baking soda in an eight-ounce cup of lukewarm bottled water (without chlorine) and dispensing it from a spray bottle. You can also use sea salt without iodine. Spray into each nostril while closing off the other nostril and simultaneously inhaling. This is nonaddictive and can be done as often as you like throughout the day. It has no negative side effects, except for the curious looks you will get from those wanting to know what you are spraying in your nose.

The *Sinus Survival Spray,* a botanical saline nasal mist, has been a highly effective addition to the Sinus Survival Program. Formulated by Dr. Steve Morris, a naturopathic physician from Mukilteo, Washington, and myself, we have been using it on ourselves and recommending it to our patients for more than eight years, with excellent results. In addition to saline, which makes up the bulk of the spray, the ingredients include:

- goldenseal: acts as an antibacterial, antifungal, and anti-inflammatory
- aloe vera: has antifungal properties and relieves irritation
- grapefruit-seed extract: an excellent antifungal

The first three ingredients are all soothing and healing to the nasal mucous membranes. The Sinus Survival Spray is available in many health food stores and can also be obtained through Thriving Health Products.

An even more effective way of moisturizing is *saline irrigation.* This procedure can result in dramatic relief from pain by reducing swelling in the nasal passages, causing a reduction of pressure in the sinus, as well as helping to empty the sinus of its infected mucus. Saltwater sprays also irrigate—that is, wash out some mucus, bacteria, and dust particles—while reducing swelling. However, they don't do it as well as the following irrigation methods. Throughout the past decade I've heard many people comment that nasal irrigation, using any of the first three techniques described below, has been the *single most helpful component* of the entire Sinus Survival Program. Irrigation should be done three to four times a day for acute sinusitis and once or twice for a milder chronic condition. Many former sinus sufferers continue to irrigate daily on a preventive basis, even after curing their chronic sinusitis.

Mix the saline solution for irrigation fresh each day in one cup of lukewarm bottled water. Add one quarter to one half of a teaspoon of non-iodized table salt or sea salt and a tiny pinch of baking soda, thus making the solution close to normal body fluid salinity and pH. Irrigating with plain water is usually somewhat uncomfortable. Use the full cup of saline solution for each irrigation (one-half cup for each nostril). Lean over the sink, with the head rotated so that the nostril to be irrigated is directly above the other nostril, while using one of the following methods. Always blow your nose *very gently* after irrigating.

Method 1
For the past seven years I have been recommending the use of the Neti Pot, and more recently SinuCleanse, for nasal irrigation. It is a small porcelain pot with a narrow spout (SinuCleanse is plastic with a very similar shape and size). This is probably the most gentle and convenient method for irrigation. Because of this, people with chronic sinusitis are much more apt to use this method on a regular basis, both therapeutically in treating an infection and preventively. SinuCleanse is sold with packets of hypertonic saline to mix with water, making this method even more convenient. The Neti Pot is made by the Himalayan Institute in Honesdale, Pennsylvania, and is available in many health food stores. SinuCleanse is available through Thriving Health Products.

Method 2

Use an angled nasal irrigator attachment (the Grossan nasal irrigator is available at some pharmacies) on a Water Pik appliance. Set the Water Pik at the *lowest* possible pressure and insert the irrigator tip just inside one nostril, pinching your nostril to form a seal. Irrigate with your mouth open, allowing the fluid to drain out either your mouth or nose. Repeat the procedure in the other nostril. The pulsations of the Water Pik make this perhaps the most effective method for irrigation. However, it is also the most expensive.

Method 3

Completely fill a large, all-rubber ear syringe (available at most pharmacies) with saline solution. Lean over the sink and insert the syringe tip just inside one nostril, so that it forms a comfortable seal. *Gently* squeeze and release the bulb several times to swish the solution around the inside of your nose. The solution will run out both nostrils and may also run out of your mouth. Repeat this for each nostril until one cup of saline solution is used, or until the solution is clear.

Method 4

For very small children, irrigate with ten to twenty drops of saline solution per nostril from an eyedropper.

If you are using a decongestant nasal spray or a corticosteroid nasal spray, use them only *after* the saltwater nasal irrigations.

These methods obviously require more effort than the saline nasal sprays, but many patients comment on how much more helpful it is.

Another solution that has been effective in irrigation is called Alkalol. It is a mucus solvent and cleaner, and can be used with the saline solution in a 1:1 ratio (one-half saline, one-half Alkalol) with all of the methods previously mentioned. You will probably have to ask your pharmacist to order it for you, as it is not usually available, but Alkalol is very inexpensive.

Water, moisture, and nasal hygiene—that is, saline spray, steam, and irrigation—can also help to relieve the symptoms of dry, crusted nasal membranes that are common with chronic sinusitis and often prone to nosebleeds. You can apply Neosporin ointment or even better Ponaris nasal emollient (ask your pharmacist to order it) to the nasal membranes twice daily with a Q-Tip or your little finger.

3. Food and Supplements
DIET

Food and supplements are the third of the *essential 8*. The foods listed below in the *Headache Relief Diet* have all been identified as possible triggers for *migraine* headache, *tension* headache, and many can also trigger a *cluster* headache during a cluster cycle. For migraine, I recommend that you eliminate all of these foods for at least a month (for cluster, eliminate them during a cluster cycle), and then gradually, every 3 to 4 days, reintroduce one of the foods from the list. This food *elimination diet* will help you determine if a particular food is one of your headache triggers. The most common triggers for cluster headache (only during the cluster cycle) include alcohol, and nitrites found in aged cheeses, aged meats, chocolate, and MSG, a common food additive. In addition to all of the well-known migraine triggers listed in the Headache Relief Diet, there are a number of other foods to which migraineurs might be sensitive. The most common documented food sensitivities have been shown to be: cow's milk, wheat, rye, corn, orange, eggs, tomato, beef, pork, yeast, shellfish, peanuts, coffee, tea, and chocolate. A food-elimination trial should also include this entire list. You may experience significant improvement from migraine simply as a result of this diet. In addition to identifying and avoiding migraine triggers and food sensitivities, another preventive dietary measure would be to decrease fats from land-based animals and to increase foods that inhibit platelet aggregation (thus preventing release of serotonin). These foods include vegetable oils—flax oil and olive oil, onion, garlic, and fish oils. Since free radicals contribute to migraines, it is important to eat more whole foods that are high in antioxidant vitamins and minerals (see page 128). The same is true for tension headaches. Stress depletes the body of micronutrients, the most important of which are the antioxidant vitamins C, E, beta-carotene, B complex, and the minerals calcium, magnesium, potassium, zinc, manganese, and selenium. A megadose multivitamin-mineral product can easily meet all of these needs.

HEADACHE RELIEF DIET

FOODS TO AVOID

I. **High Tyramine-Containing Foods**
  A. Ripened cheeses
    Blue, Boursault, brick (natural), Brie, Camembert, cheddar, Emmentaler, Gruyère, mozzarella, Parmesan, Romano, Roquefort, Stilton
    Permissible cheeses are: American, Velveeta, cottage cheese, and cream cheese
  B. Aged meat and fish
    Liver, caviar, pickled herring, fermented sausage (bologna, pepperoni, salami, summer sausage), and processed meat (hot dogs and ham)
  C. Alcoholic Beverages
    Red wine (chianti in particular), beer, sherry
  D. Vegetables
    Sauerkraut, pods of broad beans (string, lima, pinto, garbanzo, and navy beans; and peas)
  E. Fruits
    Avocados (especially if overrripe, i.e., guacamole), figs (especially canned), citrus fruit (no more than one serving per day: one orange or grapefruit, or one glass of orange juice), bananas (especially if overripe), papayas, raisins
  F. Any fermented, pickled, or marinated food
    Vinegar (especially red wine vinegar), yogurt, sour cream, buttermilk, soy, yeast extracts, brewer's yeast, and sourdough bread

II. **Foods That Dilate the Blood Vessels and Therefore Can Precipitate a Vascular Headache**
   A. All alcoholic beverages—If you must drink, the following are recommended: Seagram's V.O., Cutty Sark, Haute Sauterne Riesling, vodka.
   B. Monosodium glutamate (MSG)—May be identified on food labels as hydrolyzed vegetable protein, natural flavoring, or seasoning. Found in Chinese foods, canned soups, frozen dinners, Accent, Lawry's Seasoning Salt, Hamburger Helper, etc. Check labels of all canned and packaged foods
   C. NutraSweet (aspartame)
   D. Nitrites
      Hot dogs, turkey dogs, chicken dogs, bacon
   E. Excessive amounts of niacin (niacinamide is fine) and vitamin A (over 25,000 IU daily).

III. **Other Foods That Can Cause Headaches**
   A. Cow's milk, wheat, corn, orange, eggs, beef, yeast, chocolate, cane sugar, mushrooms, nuts, and seeds (sunflower, sesame, pumpkin)
   B. Caffeine (no more than two cups total per day)
      coffee, cola drinks, nonherbal teas, and some aspirin medications such as Anacin, Excedrin, and Vanquish—check labels.
   C. Raw garlic and onions (cooked are fine)
   D. Hot fresh breads, raised coffee cakes, and raised doughnuts

IV. **Eat Regularly, Don't Skip Meals**—this may result in hypoglycemia, which is another headache trigger

Reactive *hypoglycemia,* or a low blood-sugar level, was first identified as a cause of migraine headaches as long ago as 1949 in a study at the University of Michigan Medical School. Headache improvement occurs when all the refined sugar, caffeine, and alcohol is removed from your diet (although there can be temporary aggravation of symptoms when withdrawing from these substances); meals are more frequent (6 times a day); and intake of complex carbohydrates and/or protein is increased. However, *food allergy,* is a much more common migraine trigger than hypoglycemia and has been scientifically documented for more than sixty years. In a landmark study in 1979 performed by British physician, Ellen Grant, 60 patients developed migraine symptoms most frequently from the foods listed in III.A. above, in addition to tea and coffee. The average number of foods causing symptoms in each patient was ten. When the symptom-provoking foods were removed from the diet, all 60 patients improved. The number of headaches in the group fell from 402 to 6 per month, with 85 percent of the patients becoming headache-free. A secondary benefit to this study was the fact that the 15 patients who also had high blood pressure at the start of the study saw their blood pressure return to normal.

In conjunction with the Headache Relief Diet, other nutritional recommendations for migraine include decreasing fats from land animals and increasing foods that inhibit platelet aggregation, including vegetable oils, onion, garlic, fish oils. Since free radicals play a role in migraine, your diet should also emphasize whole foods with high antioxidant vitamin and mineral content.

To meet the objective of optimal health, a highly nutritious diet is essential. There is not one universal diet that ideally suits every individual. Certain lab tests (including blood type), a comprehensive nutritional history, and personal experimentation (trial and error), along with the guidance of a holistic physician, can assist you in determining the diet best suited to your unique requirements. The following guidelines, however, are self-care approaches to establishing a diet for which almost anyone can derive significant health benefits.

The importance of a healthy diet in relationship to health has been emphasized for centuries in both the East and West. While proper diet alone may not be enough to entirely reverse certain types of ailments (this is true of headache), most chronic medical conditions can be significantly improved by a diet of nutrient-rich foods and adequate intake of purified water. Unfortunately, our society, with its overreliance on fast foods and snacks, affords great temptation to stray from healthy eating habits. And even when we do resolve to change our diet for the better, many of us wind up confused about what foods to actually eat and how they should be prepared, due in great part to the steady introduction of best-selling books touting the "latest and greatest" cure-all diet. While such books may be well-intentioned, not all of them contain scientifically supported recommendations, and those that do often contradict equally researched published information that made the best-seller's list the year before. As a result, a number of polls now indicate that growing numbers of Americans are literally "fed up" with the amount of dietary and nutritional information that is becoming increasingly prevalent in our society.

A good dose of "common sense" can go a long way toward alleviating this confusion. There is a great deal of truth to the old adage "You are what you eat." The foods you consume become the fuel your body uses to carry out its countless functions. Therefore, it makes good sense to eat those foods that are the best "fuel sources." This means foods that are rich in vitamins, minerals, enzymes, essential fatty and amino acids and other necessary nutrients, free of preservatives, pesticides, and other substances that deplete the body's energy, can damage your vital organs, and fan the flames on inflammation and headache. Dr. Todd Nelson's (my coauthor of both *Arthritis* and *Asthma Survival*) recommended diet, the *New Life Eating Plan (NLEP),* is the one I follow and suggest to my patients. This diet has two components: Phase I of NLEP serves as the basis of healthy eating for those who are experiencing chronic illness and for the initial stages of rebalancing body chemistry to help restore optimal function. It is comprehensively presented in each of the two above-mentioned books. For most people with headache as their sole chronic health problem, adherence to the Headache Relief Diet and Phase II of the NLEP (presented below) will be sufficient to obtain significant improvement.

RETHINKING THE AMERICAN WAY OF EATING

In January 1992, the U.S. Department of Agriculture (USDA) unveiled its recommended dietary pyramid as a guideline for meeting these nutritional needs. (See Figure 4.5)

At the base of this pyramid are whole grains, such as brown rice, bulgur, wheat (breads and pasta), oats, barley, millet, and cereals, with a recommended 6–11 servings from this food group per day. The next section of the pyramid is divided into the categories of fruits and vegetables, with a recommended 2–4 servings of the former and 3–5 servings of the latter. Moving

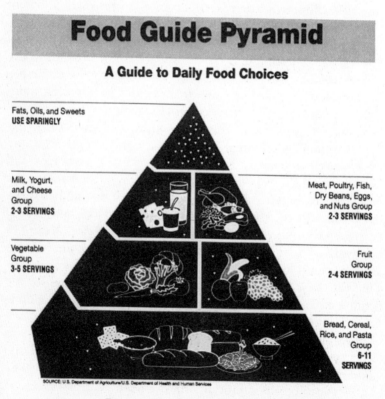

Food Guide Pyramid

A Guide to Daily Food Choices

Fats, Oils, and Sweets
USE SPARINGLY

Milk, Yogurt, and Cheese Group
2-3 SERVINGS

Meat, Poultry, Fish, Dry Beans, Eggs, and Nuts Group
2-3 SERVINGS

Vegetable Group
3-5 SERVINGS

Fruit Group
2-4 SERVINGS

Bread, Cereal, Rice, and Pasta Group
6-11 SERVINGS

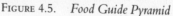

SOURCE: U.S. Department of Agriculture/U.S. Department of Health and Human Services

FIGURE 4.5.   *Food Guide Pyramid*

upward, we find a recommended 2–3 servings each of dairy products (milk, yogurt, and cheese), and the meats, poultry, fish, eggs, dry beans, and nut group. Fats, oils, and sweets, at the top of the pyramid, should be used sparingly.

While the USDA food pyramid can be a useful place to start, a number of recent studies now indicate that our daily need for carbohydrates from whole grains may not be as vital as our need for fresh fruits and vegetables. A good deal of this research has been popularized by Dr. Barry Sears, Ph.D., in his book *The Zone*. He and other researchers have found that there are a variety of harmful effects resulting from excessive intake of carbohydrates, especially those that have a high *glycemic index* (they break down quickly and release glucose into the blood at a rapid rate). These ill effects include:

- Overstimulation of insulin production, which can lead to excess storage of fat in the body, hypoglycemia, increased inflammation, cardiac risk, and diabetes.
- Diminished physical and mental capacity.
- Fluctuating energy levels and mood swings.
- Predisposition to other chronic diseases, including arthritis, heart disease, and skin disorders.

As a result, practitioners of holistic medicine now place more emphasis on the fruit and vegetable groups, recommending more servings of these two food groups over whole grains, breads, pasta, and cereal. Flour-based food—bread, pasta, and bagels—have a very high glycemic index. Whole grains, beans and legumes, and most starchy vegetables, except potatoes, have a low glycemic index and are emphasized in the NLEP. It is also recommended that milk—other than 1% or skim—be eliminated, and that your daily intake of butter, margarine, and cheese be reduced.

Table 4.2
Glycemic Index

Carbohydrates act like a powerful drug elevating insulin in the body. This in turn can increase fat deposits, LDL cholesterol (the unhealthy kind), and inflammation, while decreasing immunity. The amount of insulin the body produces is based on the amount of carbohydrates that actually enters the bloodstream as the simple sugar glucose. This is why you can consume a large amount of the 3-percent or 6-percent vegetables and fruits (refer to Table 4.3, Carbohydrate Classifications of Fruits and Vegetables, page 104) in comparison to the amount of grains, starches, breads, or pastas at any given meal.

Example: 1½ cups of broccoli, or any other 3-percent vegetable = ¼ cup pasta.

This is why it is best to focus on the low-density carbohydrates (3 percent and 6 percent). Not only can you eat more, but there are many other benefits, including high water content, high fiber content, vitamins, minerals and enzymes.

People are genetically designed to eat primarily fruits and vegetables as their major source of carbohydrates.

All carbohydrates, simple or complex, have to be broken down into simple sugars before being absorbed by the body and entering the bloodstream. The only simple sugar that can actually enter the bloodstream is glucose. The faster glucose enters the bloodstream, the more insulin you make. This is important for you to know when you are making your choice of carbohydrates. *The higher the glycemic index of carbohydrates, the faster it enters the bloodstream as sugar.*

Low Glycemic (Examples: 3-percent and 6-percent fruits and vegetables)
Fructose has to be converted into glucose via the liver, so fruits are a lower glycemic index than grains and starches.

High Glycemic (Examples: bagel, pasta, cooked starches)
Cornflakes are pure glucose linked by chemical bonds. These bonds are easily broken in the stomach and glucose rushes into the bloodstream. Table sugar is one half glucose and one half fructose, so it actually enters the bloodstream slower than a bagel.

There are other factors involved that have an effect on how fast the carbohydrates are broken down into simple sugar. Fat and soluble fibers slow the entry of glucose. Soluble fiber is an important distinction. There are two types of fiber, soluble (pectin, apples) and insoluble (cellulose and bran cereal). And because fat slows down the entry of glucose into the bloodstream, the sugar in ice cream actually is absorbed more slowly than that of a bagel. High fiber in low glycemic foods is the slowest to release sugars.

The more the carbohydrates are cooked, the higher the glycemic index will be. This is because the cell structure is broken down by cooking and processing. The glycemic index is dramatically increased in instant foods made from rice and potatoes. Therefore all bread has a high glycemic index.

Highest Glycemic Index Foods (Examples: puffed cereal and puffed rice cakes)

The body needs a constant intake of carbohydrates for optimal brain function. Too much carbohydrate and the body increases insulin secretion to drive down blood sugar. Too little and the brain will not function efficiently. (High glycemic food should always be avoided with candida overgrowth.)

Remember, protein stimulates glucagon, which reduces insulin secretion, while fat and fiber slow down the rate of entry of any carbohydrate.

BEYOND THE USDA FOOD PYRAMID

Dr. Nelson developed the NLEP after realizing that all of his chronically ill patients were making at least six critical dietary mistakes. These six are the first six on the list that he identified as the fifteen most common mistakes in the American diet that undermine health. They are:

1. Excess saturated fat, trans fats, cooked fats, and insufficient essential fatty acids (EFAs)
2. Excess sweets
3. Excess refined carbohydrates and insufficient complex carbohydrates

Table 4.3 Carbohydrate Classifications of Fruits and Vegetables
(According to Carbohydrate Content)

VEGETABLES

3%	6%	15%	20+%
asparagus	beans, string	artichoke	beans, dried
bean sprouts	beets	carrot	beans, lima
beet greens	brussels sprouts	oyster plant	corn
broccoli	chives	parsnip	potato, sweet
cabbage	collard greens	peas, green	potato, white
cauliflower	dandelion greens	squash	yam
celery	eggplant		
chard, swiss	kale		
cucumber	kohlrabi		
endive	leek		
lettuce	okra		
mustard greens	onion		
radish	parsley		
spinach	pepper, red		
watercress	pimento		
	pumpkin		
	rutabagas		
	turnip		

FRUITS

3%	6%	15%	20+%
cantaloupe	apricot (fresh only)	apple	banana
melons	blackberries	grapes	figs
rhubarb	blueberries	kumquats	prunes
strawberries	cherries	loganberries	or any dried
tomato	cranberries	mango	fruit
	grapefruit	mulberries	watermelon
	guava	pear	
	kiwi	pineapple (fresh)	
	lemon	pomegranate	
	lime		
	melons		
	orange		
	papaya		
	peach		
	plum		
	raspberries		
	tangerine		

4. Excess alcohol
5. Excess caffeine
6. Excess salt
7. Excess consumption of overly cooked food
8. Excess processed and devitalized food
9. Excess "high-stress" protein sources and insufficient "low-stress" protein sources
10. Excess consumption of foodborne toxins (preservatives, additives, artificial sweeteners, colorings, flavoring, hydrogenated fats)
11. Insufficient high-quality, fresh organic produce—both fruits and vegetables
12. Insufficient pure water
13. Insufficient balanced fiber intake
14. Poor food combinations
15. Stressful eating environment and insufficient chewing

Consistently making poor choices in these fifteen areas over the course of a lifetime will usually result in poor health. This occurs from the cumulative effect of increased chemical toxicity, free-radical damage, nutrient depletion, and dysbiosis resulting in immune, endocrine, neurologic, rheumatologic, and cardiac dysfunction.

Dr. Nelson has concluded that the goal of any dietary program for preventing and treating a chronic illness, including headache, should be targeted at correcting these common mistakes and establishing a regenerative way of eating for life. This is the primary purpose of the New Life Eating Plan. As you begin to adopt these principles, you'll soon realize that this diet is an essential component of the daily practice of loving and nurturing yourself.

Let's now explore some of the specific steps you can take in committing to the NLEP or a comparably healthy diet. Out of the fifteen most common mistakes, we will emphasize changing the first six on the list above. These are perhaps the most important mistakes that we commonly make, which we refer to as "The Sickening Six."

THE SICKENING SIX

There are six substances in the American diet that should be substantially eliminated—unhealthy fats, sugar, refined carbohydrates, alcohol, caffeine, and salt. These "sickening six" can lead to a variety of disease conditions. While it is all right to enjoy these substances in moderation, keeping their intake to a minimum can pay big health dividends. Here are a number of reasons why:

1. Unhealthy Fats

The regular intake of good fats is essential to our health. Unfortunately, most of us are getting too much unhealthy fat in our diets. Primary sources of these harmful fats include red meats, milk and other dairy products, and the hydrogenated trans fats found in margarine, cooking fats, and many brands of peanut butter. These fats are also found in many packaged foods, including most commercial cereals, which also tend to be loaded with sugar.

Unhealthy fats lead to arteriosclerosis and the buildup of plaque on the inner lining of the arteries, where over time they obstruct the flow of blood and the transport of oxygen and nutrients to the body's internal organs. This obstruction, in turn, can lead to heart attacks, angina, stroke, kidney failure, and pre-gangrene in the legs.

The excessive intake of unhealthy fats are also associated with certain cancers. Among them are cancer of the breast, colon, rectum, prostate, ovaries, and uterus. This is particularly true of the saturated fats derived from meat products.

Obesity, which is increasing to epidemic proportions in this country, is also directly related to excessive fat (and sugar) intake. Obesity is a serious disease condition by itself, but if prolonged, it can contribute to many other forms of illness, including adult-onset diabetes.

Becoming aware of your fat intake and minimizing the amount of harmful fats you consume is an important step toward optimal health.

2. Sugar

The use of sugar in your diet can pose many harmful health risks, yet the average American consumes 150 pounds each year. This is the equivalent of over 40 teaspoons of sugar every day. The following are only a few of sugar's health-depleting effects:

• Sugar has been shown to be a risk factor for heart disease, *and may be more harmful than fat.*
• Sugar weakens the immune system, increasing susceptibility to infection and allergy, and further exacerbating all other diseases caused by diminished immune function.
• Sugar stimulates excessive insulin production, thereby causing more fat to be stored in the body; lowers HDL cholesterol levels (the healthy cholesterol); increases the production of harmful triglycerides; and increases the risk of arteriosclerosis (hardening of the arteries).
• Sugar contributes to diminished mental capacity and can cause feelings of anxiety, depression, and rage. It has also been implicated in certain cases of attention deficit disorder (ADD).
• High sugar intake is associated with certain cancers, including cancer of the gallbladder and colon. Recently, sugar has also been implicated as a causative factor in cases of breast cancer.
• Excessive sugar in the diet is a primary contributor to candidiasis (intestinal yeast overgrowth), which can lead to a host of health problems, including gastrointestinal disorders, asthma, bronchitis, sinusitis, allergies, and chronic fatigue.

If you still feel a need to satisfy your sweet tooth, substitute modest amounts of pure honey, maple syrup, or the herb Stevia, to decrease the risk of these adverse effects.

3. Refined Carbohydrates

Refined, or simple, carbohydrates, such as those found in white breads, and pastas made from white flour, are another group of health-threatening agents. When eaten to excess, these types of foods overstimulate insulin production and produce the same excessive fat storage in the body that results from eating too much sugar. This can lead to the onset of diabetes and obesity. The rise in obesity among American children is due in part to a diet heavy in sugars and refined carbohydrates, and lacking in nutritious alternatives, notably fruits and vegetables.

Several recent studies have shown that certain carbohydrates previously promoted as being "whole" sources of starch are very rapidly digested and absorbed. As a result, they elevate blood sugar fully as much as sugar itself, contributing to all of the problems cited above (see "Sugar"). Most carbohydrates have been carefully analyzed and assigned a *glycemic index* rating (for a rating of fruits and vegetables, refer to page 104). A high glycemic index indicates that a food acts much like sugar in the body, while food sources with a low glycemic index are much slower to be assimilated and therefore offer much better nutritional value. High-glycemic-index foods include: cornflakes, puffed rice, instant and mashed potatoes, white bread, maltose, and, of course, sugar itself. Foods with a low glycemic index include whole-grain cereals (oats, brown rice, amaranth, kamut, millet), legumes (beans, peas, peanuts, soybeans), pumpernickel breads, whole-wheat pastas, pearled barley, bulgur wheat, white rice, baked potatoes, sweet potatoes, apples, oranges, yogurt, and fructose (see "Glycemic Index," page 102).

4. Alcohol

Alcohol is another example of a substance that, when taken in moderation, may enhance health, but when consumed in excess can cause a variety of serious problems. And as you've also learned, even in small amounts (especially red wine and beer) it can be a headache trigger (both migraine and cluster). A growing body of research now indicates that one or two beers or a glass of wine per day can be beneficial to health as a way to relieve stress and to improve digestion. In fact, studies have shown that complete abstainers from alcohol have a slightly shorter life expectancy than those who drink in moderate amounts. Unfortunately, for many men especially, alcohol and moderation usually "don't mix."

Although most people drink in order to feel better, evidence indicates that alcohol can significantly contribute to feelings of depression, loneliness, restlessness, and boredom, according to studies conducted by the National Center for Health Statistics. In addition, very moody people are also three times as likely to be heavy drinkers (three or more drinks per day).

Aside from the social stigma surrounding excessive alcohol consumption, too much alcohol can also contribute to obesity; increased blood pressure; diabetes; colon, stomach, breast, mouth, esophageal, laryngeal, and pancreatic cancers; gastrointestinal disorders; impaired liver function; candidiasis; impaired mental functioning; and behavioral and emotional dysfunctions. If you are having difficulty in bringing your alcohol consumption under control, seek the help of a professional counselor.

5. Caffeine

Caffeine is a drug to which more than half of all Americans are addicted. On average, we drink at least two and a half cups of coffee a day, or 425 mg of caffeine. Because caffeine acts as a stimulant, we consume it in order to have more energy. But the quick-fix boost it provides usually only lasts for a few hours, leaving us with greater fatigue and irritability once its effects wear off. Typically, when this happens, we reach for another cup of coffee to keep us going. The result is a roller coaster of ups and downs that, over time, can result in a number of health hazards.

Caffeine is listed in the Headache Relief Diet as a potential headache trigger in almost any amount for those headache sufferers who are sensitive to it. For people who are regular caffeine drinkers, withdrawal from caffeine will often trigger a headache that is most effectively relieved with more caffeine. While caffeine in moderation (200 mg or less per day) is relatively safe, the regular consumption of greater amounts can result in elevated blood pressure; increased risk of cancer, heart disease, and osteoporosis; poor sleep patterns; anxiety and irritability; dizziness;

impaired circulation; urinary frequency; and gastrointestinal disorders. Caffeine also causes loss of calcium from muscle cells and can interfere with the blood-clotting process by decreasing platelet stickiness.

Taken in moderation, however, caffeine has been shown to enhance mental functioning and to improve both alertness and mood, suggesting that 200 mg or less of caffeine per day may be safely tolerated by most individuals.

If you consider yourself addicted to caffeine, the best way to break your habit is to reduce your intake *very gradually,* over a period of a few weeks or even months. Start by substituting noncaffeinated drinks, such as herbal tea or a roasted grain beverage, in place of one of your normal cups of coffee per day. Over time, cut back further while increasing the number of substitute beverages, and beware of possible withdrawal symptoms—primarily headache, in addition to nervousness and irritability. Typically, these will pass within a day or two. Also avoid other caffeine sources, such as soft drinks (particularly colas), cocoa, chocolate, and nonherbal teas.

6. Salt

Salt is another ingredient that is far too prevalent in many diets, and it poses particular dangers for certain people who suffer from high blood pressure. Many of us have been conditioned since childhood to crave salt, but its overuse draws water into the bloodstream. This, in turn, increases blood volume, causing higher blood pressure levels. Too much salt also upsets the body's sodium-potassium balance, thereby interfering with the lymphatic system's ability to draw wastes away from the cells.

Although some salt can be used in cooking, a good rule of thumb is to avoid adding salt to your food once it is served.

BEGINNING THE NLEP

As a starting point in changing your diet (you can start this either concurrent with or subsequent to the Headache Relief

Diet), reduce your intake of red meat, and when you do eat it, chose only the leanest cuts. In its place, have two to three servings per day of either fish, poultry, beans, or nuts. Also avoid all cooking fats and oils derived from animal products and those from vegetable sources that are hydrogenated and found in most margarines, many brands of peanut butter, and hydrogenated cooking fats. Instead, use vegetable oils, such as olive, or canola. Flaxseed oil, a particularly rich source of vital omega-3 essential fatty acids, can also be used (but not for cooking). The best fats are from whole vegetables and grains that are unprocessed, polyunsaturated, and non-oxidized.

Also pay attention to the various food additives that are commonly found in the typical American diet. These include all chemical preservatives, such as BHA, BHT, sodium nitrate, and sulfites; artificial coloring agents; and artificial sweeteners, such as saccharin, aspartame (NutraSweet), and cyclamates. These additives have the potential to be enormous health risks (NutraSweet can be a migraine trigger). To avoid their use, stay away from processed or canned foods and get in the habit of reading labels whenever you go shopping.

Finally, if you aren't already in the habit of doing so, consider selecting fruits and vegetables that are grown organically, and meats and poultry derived from animals that are raised free-range. In the former case, you will be eating foods that are richer in nutrients and free of pesticides, artificial fertilizers, preservatives, and other additives. Free-range meats and poultry are the end products of animals that are not subject to injections of growth hormones, antibiotics, and irradiation commonly found in meats and poultry raised commercially.

If you begin the NLEP after eliminating all of the "foods to avoid" for a full month, you are ready to expand your food choices. At this point in your Headache Survival Program, try reintroducing the list of foods you've just eliminated back into your diet. Allow them only one at a time every four to six days so you can be more aware of symptoms and track any food reactions. Score your symptoms each day on the Symptom Chart. If your symptoms seem to increase within a 24-to-72-hour period, and you haven't made any other significant dietary changes, then you are probably reacting to that new food and should continue to avoid it. If you are unsure, keep that food out of your diet for 7 days and retest it.

Once you know you can tolerate a food, allow it on a rotational basis, which means one time every 3 to 5 days. For example, if you have cheese on Monday, wait until Thursday to have it again so your body has a chance to clear any reactions it may have to it. This also helps you to prevent developing a reaction to that specific food. But be careful! Many people will experience great results from eating like this and then adopt the attitude "I've been doing well, so now I can go back to some of the old foods that I love." In fact, you might be tempted to go overboard in the opposite direction. The worst that can happen is that you will begin to experience more frequent headaches. This is simply your body wisely reminding you to get back to a healthy diet. Let's now look at a safe, gradual way to expand your choices, while continuing to eliminate headache triggers, minimize toxicity and allergic reactions, and maximize nutrient density.

Foods to Test Rotating Back into Your Diet
(These are foods to generally deemphasize in the diet and are not required to be healthy. They should only be allowed back in if you enjoy them and you continue to feel well while eating them.)

Cheese—all types
Cultured dairy—nonfat yogurt or cottage cheese
Citrus fruit
Meat and fish
Wheat
Corn
Beans and legumes—if not already eating them
Whole-grain rye crackers
Higher-glycemic foods: flour-based foods such as whole-grain
    pasta, bread, pancakes, muffins, starchier fruits, and vegetables

Small amounts of sweetener: Stevia is best, or honey, maple syrup, brown rice syrup.

Remember: It's what you do most of the time—day in and day out—with your diet that counts. Maintain a lot of variety so you won't get bored. Do the best you can. Your headache symptoms will let you know if you need to do better.

What follow, by category, are listings of a variety of nutritious foods that can be added to your diet for their rich nutrient value.

Fruits and Vegetables

Fresh fruits and vegetables, organic when possible, should be a staple of your daily diet. Not only are they rich with nutrients, they also possess vital cleansing properties and high-fiber content that helps rid the body of waste and toxins, creating greater levels of energy. Be sure to eat at least part of your daily servings of fruits and vegetables raw, since in this form you will be receiving the highest nutrient content. Lightly steaming vegetables is another healthy way to prepare them. Boiling or overcooking vegetables, on the other hand, can destroy the abundant vitamins, minerals, and enzymes in these foods.

Among the fruits and vegetables with the greatest nutritional value (especially vitamin C and carotenes) are: oranges, cantaloupe, strawberries, apples, guavas, red chili peppers, red and green sweet peppers, kale, parsley, greens (mustard, collard, and turnip), broccoli, cauliflower, brussels sprouts, carrots, yams, spinach, mangoes, winter squash, romaine lettuce, asparagus, tomatoes, onions, garlic, mushrooms, peaches, papayas, bananas, cherries, grapefruit, watermelon, grapes, plums, blueberries, and sprouts. **NOTE:** *Although they are extremely rich sources of vitamins, minerals, and fiber, fruits impede the digestion of other foods and are therefore best eaten separately from meals.*

Whole Grains and Complex Carbohydrates

Whenever possible, whole grains, beans, and legumes should be your primary source of carbohydrates, as they, too, provide many essential vitamins and minerals. Most grains also supply about 10 percent of excellent-quality protein. Among the recommended whole grains are: amaranth, millet, brown rice, basmati rice, quinoa, barley, rye, and oats. Use wheat sparingly on a rotation basis, according to NLEP Phase II. Other sources of complex carbodyrates are starchy vegetables and legumes. Complex carbohydrates provide sustained boosts of energy and digest slowly, releasing their sugars into the bloodstream gradually. This gradual release of sugars helps to maintain insulin balance and contributes to the production of *adenosine triphosphate* (ATP) in the cells, thereby strengthening the immune system. Good sources of starchy vegetables include: sweet potatoes, yams, acorn and butternut squash, and pumpkins. For legumes, choose black beans, garbanzo beans (chick peas), lima beans, aduki beans, navy beans, kidney beans, lentils, black-eyed peas, or split peas.

Proteins

Proteins are the nutrients your body uses to build cells, repair tissue, and produce the basic building blocks of DNA and RNA. Bones, hair, nails, muscle fibers, collagen, and other connective tissues are all composed of protein, and protein itself is second only to water in terms of the body's overall composition.

The main sources of protein for a healthy diet are: fish, chicken, and turkey (select cuts that are free-range and free of hormones and antibiotics), healthy eggs, soy products (soy milk, tofu, miso, and tempeh), sunflower seeds, almonds, cashews, pine nuts, pecans, walnuts, raw pumpkin seeds, and sesame seeds. Red meats and dairy products are not on this list because of their higher concentration of unhealthy fats, which can contribute to a host of disease conditions, especially heart disease and hardening of the arteries, and inflammation. Low-fat or nonfat cultured dairy products, such as yogurt and cottage cheese, are well tolerated by many people.

Fats and Oils

Contrary to popular belief, all of us need a certain amount of fat in our diet. Fats supply energy reserves that the body draws upon when not enough fat is present in the foods we eat. Fats also serve as a primary form of insulation and help to maintain normal body temperature. In addition, fats help to transport oxygen; absorb fat-soluble vitamins (A, D, E, and K); nourish the skin, mucous membranes, and nerves; and serve as an anti-inflammatory. Healthy fat is utilized by the body in the form of essential fatty acids (EFAs).

Excessive fat intake, however, can contribute to a variety of illnesses, especially obesity and heart disease. Fat intake that is too low can also pose health risks. One of the keys to optimal health, then, is to make sure that you are getting an adequate supply of fats in your diet, and that they are "good" fats, not fats that are harmful. These good fats, in the form of oils, remain liquid at room temperature.

The best food sources of healthy fats are the whole foods from which the oils are derived. These include foods such as nuts and seeds, soybeans, olives, avocados, and wheat germ. Healthy fats in the form of oils include: olive, canola, flaxseed (do not use for cooking), and sesame. Essential fatty acids are found predominantly in two groups, the omega-3s and the omega-6s. Good sources of omega-3 include cold-water fish (salmon, sardines, tuna, sole), wild game, flaxseeds and flaxseed oil, canola oil, walnuts, pumpkin seeds, soybeans, fresh sea vegetables, and leafy greens. Good sources of omega-6 include vegetable oils, legumes, all nuts and seeds, and most grains, breast milk, organ meats, lean meats, leafy greens, borage oil, evening primrose oil, gooseberry, and black currant oils.

Fiber

Fiber is one of the most overlooked components of a healthy diet, with the average American diet supplying only one-fourth to one-third of the amount necessary for optimal health. High-fiber diets are associated with less coronary heart disease, lower cholesterol and triglyceride levels, lower blood pressure, lower incidence of cancer (especially colon and rectum), better control of diabetes, and lower incidences of diverticulitis, appendicitis, gallbladder disease, ulcerative colitis, and hernias. Lack of fiber is also the major cause of constipation and hemorrhoids.

Fiber includes the nondigestible substances in the foods that we eat. Good sources of fiber include fruits; the bran portion of whole grains, such as whole wheat, rolled oats, and brown rice; and raw and cooked green, yellow, and starchy vegetables, such as spinach, romaine lettuce, squash, carrots, beans, and lentils. The goal is 25–35 grams of fiber intake per day.

Vitamins, Minerals, and Herbs

In this section most of the products I recommend are available in health food stores, and some are only available through Thriving Health Products (1-888-434-0033).

MIGRAINE HEADACHE

Herbs

Feverfew (*Tanacetum parthenium*) is a medicinal herb with a long history (in England) of treating migraines and arthritis. It is the only herbal remedy for migraine studied in double-blind fashion. In a survey of 270 individuals with migraines who had taken feverfew every day for prolonged periods of time, more than 70 percent believed the herb decreased the frequency and/or severity of their attacks. Seventeen of those who had seen a positive response to feverfew then participated in a double-blind study, in which they were either continued on feverfew or given a placebo. Those taking the placebo became significantly worse, with increases in the frequency and severity of headaches, naud vomiting. In contrast, those who continued on feverfew ned their previous improvement.

Feverfew is considered moderately effective for preventing migraine, and is not recommended for treating an attack. Therefore, it needs to be taken regularly over a long period. It is rich in compounds known as sesquiterpine lactones, of which 85 percent consist of the compound *parthenolide*. This is the substance that benefits migraineurs by helping to control the expansion and contraction of blood vessels in the brain. Several studies have shown that parthenolide inhibits platelet (a blood component involved with clotting) aggregation and the release of serotonin (the dominant neurotransmitter in migraine) from platelets and polymorphonuclear leukocyte (white blood cells) granules. It also inhibits inflammatory prostaglandin synthesis and the release of arachidonic acid (causes inflammation). There is one other study besides the one just described, also placebo-controlled, showing that feverfew causes a significant reduction in pain intensity as well as in the associated symptoms of nausea. The dose of feverfew varies according to the preparation used, but can range from 5 mg per day of dried leaves to 120 mg of standardized extract containing no less than 0.2% parthenolide. The typical dosage is 0.25 to 0.5 mg pathenolide 2 times per day. Aphthous ulcers (canker sores) and GI (gastrointestinal) tract disturbances may occur occasionally, especially when migraineurs chew the raw leaves. Feverfew is a member of the *Compositae* (Asterace) family, and people allergic to plants in this family, such as chamomile or ragweed, should not take feverfew. Anyone using anticoagulants should not take feverfew because of the platelet inhibition activity with increased risk of bleeding. Feverfew is also contraindicated in pregnancy. It is a relatively inexpensive herb.

Butterbur extract: Found within a product called Petadolex.

Ginger (*Zingiber officinale*) is another useful herb in treating migraine and especially the nausea that often accompanies a migraine attack. Ginger has chemicals that act as natural COX-2 inhibitors to reduce pain and inflammation. It is a digestive aid that soothes and relaxes the intestinal tract. Dried or powdered ginger in a dosage of 500 mg 4 times a day has been shown to be effective. Although no studies support it, some migraineurs have reported that 500 mg of powdered ginger at the first sign of a migraine will abort the headache.

Ginkgo biloba 40 to 60 mg 3 times a day and **Pueraria root** have also been used for treating migraine.

It may be surprising to learn that **Cannabis sativa** and its relative, *Cannabis indica,* were once widely accepted medical treatments for the prevention and relief of migraine headache, and were listed in the *United States Pharmacopeia* from 1860 to 1941. Despite vigorous protest by the American Medical Association, *Cannabis* was made illegal in the United States in 1937 and finally dropped from the *Pharmacopeia* in 1941. Sir William Osler, the acknowledged father of modern medicine, stated of migraine treatment near the turn of the twentieth century, "*Cannabis indica* is probably the most satisfactory remedy."

Although no modern clinical studies have specifically investigated the use of *Cannabis* in migraine, a number of small pain-relief studies have reported positive results in chronic headache pain and improvement of pain tolerance. The analgesic properties of *Cannabis* are believed to be a result of interference with pain transmission in the midbrain—the area of migraine generation. This recent research is particularly germane to the current controversy regarding legalizing the medicinal use of marijuana.

Vitamins

Riboflavin (vitamin B_2) has been shown to be an effective prophylactic agent. It increases mitochondrial (the mitochondria are the intracellular "power plants") energy and efficiency. A randomized placebo-controlled study performed by J. Schoenen, M.D., et al., published in *Neurology* in 1998, showed that 400 mg of riboflavin taken daily for three months effectively reduced migraine attack frequency and headache days by two-thirds. Migraine severity was reduced by 68 percent. Migraineurs should take the riboflavin for at least three months to see effectiveness. Riboflavin is well-tolerated and without significant side effects. However, since 400 mg is more than 200 times the Recommended Dietary Allowance (RDA), after relief has been obtained and you're eating a more nutritious diet, it is advisable to gradually reduce the dosage to 100 mg as a maintenance dose and see what happens with your headache symptoms. There are no long-term studies demonstrating the safety of daily doses as large as 400 mg. You can also boost your levels of riboflavin by eating more foods with high levels of this vitamin (after ruling them out as headache triggers), such as milk, eggs, meat, poultry, fish, and leafy green vegetables.

Intravenous injection of *folic acid* 15 mg in one study achieved total relief of an acute migraine within 1 hour in 60 percent of subjects, with great improvement in another 30 percent.

Vitamin B$_6$, 25 mg 3 times a day, is helpful for migraine. You can take the 75 mg of B$_6$ as part of a *vitamin B-complex. Vitamin D,* 400 IU daily, is also recommended.

The *antioxidants* (substances that prevent oxidation of cell membranes and thereby prevent cell damage), *vitamin C* 1,000 to 6,000 mg per day, in an ascorbate form or ester C; *vitamin A* or *beta-carotene* 10,000 to 25,000 IU per day; and *vitamin E* 400 to 800 IU per day, have demonstrated benefits in treating migraine. The federal government's Institute of Medicine's April 2000 guidelines on recommended daily dosages for vitamins suggests a maximum of 2,000 mg per day of C. The primary risk mentioned for megadoses of vitamin C was diarrhea. Although the Headache Survival dosages may exceed these limits, using an ascorbate form of C or ester C reduces the possibilty of these adverse side effects since they are much better tolerated in the bowel than ascorbic acid (the most common form of vitamin C). If diarrhea does occur, you can simply reduce the dosage. I personally have been taking an average of 6,000 mg of vitamin C daily for the past fifteen years without any problems whatsoever. In fact, I'm healthier than I've ever been and so are most of my patients, the majority of whom also exceed the recommended maximum daily dose of vitamin C. Linus Pauling, a two-time Nobel Prize winner who did much of the original research on the therapeutic benefits of vitamin C, took 10,000 mg daily and died at the age of ninety-three.

Minerals

Magnesium has been used with great success to both prevent and to treat migraines. Several studies have shown that many migraineurs have low levels of intracellular magnesium. It is effective in preventing migraine chiefly because of its ability to maintain cerebral blood vessel tone. Magnesium can support vascular tone by several mechanisms, including (1) inhibition of platelet aggregation; (2) interference with synthesis, release, and action of inflammatory mediators; (3) direct alterations of cerebrovascular tone; (4) inhibition of vasospasm; and (5) stabilization of cell membranes. Several studies have shown that magnesium at a dose of 400 to 600 mg per day may reduce headache frequency as well as number of days with migraine. *Magnesium-rich foods* include brown rice, popcorn, broccoli, peas, potatoes, shrimp, clams, green vegetables, and skim milk. Magnesium appears to be helpful in preventing migraine and is often effective for menstrual migraine, while intravenous magnesium can produce rapid and dramatic results in treating acute migraines. Alan Gaby, M.D., a past president of the American Holistic Medical Association and an authority on nutritional medicine, has used an intravenous combination of magnesium, calcium, B vitamins, and vitamin C (administered over 10 minutes) to successfully relieve a migraine attack, frequently within 1 or 2 minutes. One study has shown that 1 gram of IV magnesium sulfate administered to 40 consecutive patients with migraine provided very good and sustained relief of their headache. Magnesium glycinate is currently regarded as the most effective form in which to take oral magnesium.

Calcium, 1,000 mg per day, is recommended for migraine prevention, especially for menstrual migraines. It can also be used intravenously for treating acute migraine.

Supplements

Omega-3 fish oils (EPA and DHA), essential fatty acids, have been shown in one study to greatly reduce intensity and frequency of migraines. The therapeutic dosage used in the study was 14 grams daily in divided doses. However, I recommend the following: EPA (eicosapentaenoic acid) in a dosage of up to 300 mg 3×/day and DHA (docosahexaenoic acid), up to 200 mg 3×/day for 12 weeks, then reduce to 2×/day. In addition, take flaxseed oil, 1 tablespoon 2×/day with meals or 3 capsules 3×/day with meals. These essential fatty acids help reduce the pain of migraine through their action as a powerful anti-inflammatory. Seeds, nuts, cold-water fish (salmon, tuna, halibut, mackerel), and especially flaxseed oil, are all good sources of omega-3.

There has been one study suggesting that **gamma linolenic acid—GLA** (a primary ingredient of omega-6 fatty acids)— may be effective in migraine prevention. Performed by Wagner et al., and published in *Cephalgia* in 1997, polyunsaturated fatty acids consisting of 1,800 mg of gamma linolenic acid and ALA (alpha linoleic acid) were administered to 168 patients over a six-month period in an open, uncontrolled study. Eighty-six percent experienced a reduction in severity, frequency, and duration of migraine attacks. Good dietary sources of omega-6 fatty acids are safflower, sunflower, soybean, and especially evening primrose oil. A therapeutic dose of evening primrose oil is 500 mg 2 to 4 times a day.

The nutrient **5-hydroxytryptophan,** or **5-HTP,** is a derivative of the amino acid tryptophan. A mood-enhancing chemical, it has recently been demonstrated to increase pain tolerance and may also boost the brain's serotonin levels. When used long-term, 5-HTP is effective in prevention and in reducing the intensity, frequency, and duration of migraine. The recommended dosage is either 200 mg 3 times or 300 mg 2 times a day.

The supplement **S-adenosylmethionine,** or **SAM-e,** well known for treating arthritis, has also been successfully used for migraine. It has also been used for treating depression and strengthening the liver. SAM-e is produced by every cell in the body and is part of a biochemical process that helps to regulate hormones and mood-altering neurotransmitters. It contributes to the production of the amino acids cysteine and taurine, and the potent antioxidant glutathione. One of the best studies on its analgesic properties was performed on arthritics and compared SAM-e to naproxen (Aleve and Naprosyn) 750 mg per day. It was found to provide just as much pain relief. The dosage for migraine is 400 mg, 4 times per day, but you should begin with 200 mg twice daily and gradually increase over a 3-week period to the maintenance dose. It is quite safe, with possible minimal stomach distress. A positive side effect of SAM-e is that it can act as an effective antidepressant. However, SAM-e should not be combined with antidepressant medications.

Aromatherapy

Alan Hirsch, M.D., director of the Smell & Taste Treatment and Research Foundation in Chicago, studied fifty patients with migraine and found that the scent of *green apples* made headache pain fade. Migraine pain was found to improve more during an attack when the subjects sniffed tubes containing a green apple smell than when sniffing unscented tubes. Dr. Hirsch found that the specific smell of green apples reduced anxiety.

Another option for aromatherapy is to breathe from a facial steamer after adding a couple of drops of pure peppermint oil. The steam inhaler, which has been an integral part of the Sinus Survival Program for years, is excellent for steaming. Peppermint oil is available at most health food stores.

TENSION HEADACHE

Herbs

If anxiety and stress are the primary contributors to causing your headache, then both **valerian** and **kava kava** are good choices. They can be taken as tinctures, teas, or in capsules. The dosage of valerian capsules is 150 to 300 mg 3 times a day, and in tincture form, 4 to 6 ml 3 times a day. Kava kava can be taken 100 mg 3 times a day in capsules or 1 to 2 ml 3 times a day of the extract. These two herbs can be taken alone or combined with synergistic-acting herbs such as *passionflower, skullcap,* or *hops.* If no relief occurs within an hour, repeat the dose.

White willow bark (*Salix alba*), one of the original plant sources for aspirin before it was chemically synthesized, can be taken as a strong tea (up to 3 cups a day) or in capsule form (2 or 3 capsules three or four times a day).

An antispasmodic herbal preparation, **Herbal Muscle Relief** or **Herbal Muscle Relief P.M.** (a Thriving Health Product) is highly effective for treating tension headache. The product contains magnesium, calcium, and the herbs: valerian and passionflower in Herbal Muscle Relief, and valerian, passionflower, kava kava, and hops in Herbal Muscle Relief P.M. The latter is recommended for sleep. Dosage varies for prevention (2 tabs morning and night) or for pain relief (2 tabs every 3 hours).

Inflavonoid Intensive Care is a powerful combination of anti-inflammatory herbs—boswellia, curcumin, and ginger—that is just as effective an analgesic as most NSAIDs, but without the potential gastrointestinal side effects. It is COX-2 inhibiting, reduces pro-inflammatory prostaglandins, and increases anti-inflammatory prostaglandins. It is made by Metagenics and is available through Thriving Health Products. The dose recommended is 2 tabs every 3–4 hours for acute headache; 1–2 tabs morning and night is a good preventive dose.

A liquid preparation of *capsaicin* (cayenne) used intranasally has significant research-backed success for tension and *cluster* headache.

Minerals

Magnesium is probably useful for preventing tension headaches, although there are no studies to support this. A dosage of 500 mg a day of magnesium glycinate is recommended, not only for headache prevention but as part of an optimal program of dietary supplements.

Aromatherapy

A double-blind study of healthy volunteers with tension headaches showed that an external (to the temples and forehead) application of **peppermint oil** raises pain threshold and has strong relaxing effects, while **eucalyptus oil** has calming and relaxing effects and improves cognitive performance without any analgesic effect. Another study on tension headache sufferers using peppermint oil showed positive results. The oils, 5 to 10 drops of each 2 to 3 times a day, were applied to the temples and forehead and relaxed the scalp muscles. **Rosemary oil** (1 part oil to 10 of vegetable oil) massaged into the temples and forehead has also been successfully used for tension headache.

CLUSTER HEADACHE

Two of the above recommendations can also be used for treating cluster headache—**magnesium** glycinate and intranasal **capsaicin.** In addition, the following therapies have provided benefit to sufferers of cluster headache:

Melatonin—6 to 10 mg nightly, only under medical supervision, may improve daily cluster headaches within 4 to 5 days

Oxygen—100 percent oxygen at a flow of 7 liters per minute by face mask for 15 to 20 minutes while sitting

Hepataplex—a traditional Chinese herbal compound for relief of "liver heat rising" (a cause of cluster headaches); relieving liver congestion and improving bile flow can help cluster headaches (a Metagenics product)

Hot shower massager—apply with moderate pressure to the scalp.

Apply **ice** or **heat** to the area of pain—whichever one feels better.

Nutritional Supplements

I believe that you can, by taking some simple and inexpensive measures, extend your life and your years of well-being. My most important recommendation is that you take vitamins every day to optimum amounts, to supplement the vitamins you receive in your food.

—LINUS PAULING, Ph.D., two-time Nobel Prize laureate,
who lived a full and productive ninety-three years
by following his own advice.

Adhering to the dietary, herbal, mineral, vitamin, and supplement recommendations outlined above is a vital first step in improving your headaches and in creating optimal health for yourself and your loved ones. Sadly, however, a healthy diet alone or in conjunction with a few specific dietary supplements for treating headaches, even one that is rich with pure, organically grown foods, is no longer enough to ensure total physical well-being. Due to our unhealthy environment (see below) and the stresses of daily life, most of us also need to regularly supplement our diets in a more comprehensive fashion. On a daily basis we are exposed to stress in the form of chemicals, emotions, and infection. Chemical stress may come from polluted air and water, food pesticides, insecticides, heavy metals, and even radioactive wastes. More than ever before, foreign chemicals can be found in our foods and environment. Many of these are commercially synthesized, but quite a few are naturally occurring, as well. In 1989, the *Kellogg Report* stated that 1,000 newly synthesized compounds are introduced into our environment every year. That's the equivalent of three new chemicals per day. Currently, there are approximately 100,000 of these foreign chemicals, or *xenobiotics,* in the world. They include drugs, pesticides, industrial chemicals, food additives and preservatives, and environmental pollutants. As a result, it's very easy for toxic chemicals to find their way into our bodies via the air we breathe, the foods we eat, and the water we drink. We also ingest these chemicals whenever we use drugs (both medicinal and illicit), alcohol, or tobacco. How many of these might be contributing to your headaches?

Compounding this problem is the fact that the soil in which our foods are grown is greatly depleted of the trace minerals needed to create and maintain health. Many of our foods are shipped, frozen, stored, and warehoused, reaching us weeks or months after being harvested. Degeneration of their nutrient value occurs at each stop. Cooking methods, such as boiling and frying, also contribute to nutrient loss once the food reaches our kitchens and restaurants. Moreover, the standard American diet has become increasingly devoid of nutrients and overburdened with empty calories and nonfood additives. Therefore, even though the body is marvelously designed to eliminate toxins, in today's environment it needs help in doing so.

FREE RADICALS AND ANTIOXIDANTS

One of the biggest threats to our health are free radicals, highly toxic molecules that play a causative role in many disease conditions besides headaches, particularly degenerative disorders such as arthritis, heart disease, cancer, cataracts, macular degeneration, high blood pressure, emphysemia, cirrhosis of the liver, ulcers, toxemia during pregnancy, and mental disorders. Free radicals, or oxidants, are very unstable and highly reactive molecules that contain one or more unpaired electrons. They try to capture electrons off other molecules to gain stability, a process known as oxidation. They also increase susceptibility to infection and accelerate the aging process by damaging the cells.

Since free radicals are the primary agents of most cellular damage, minimizing their harmful effects is important. Antioxidants are substances that significantly delay or inhibit oxidation. They neutralize free radicals by supplying electrons. Fortunately, our bodies manufacture antioxidant enzymes within the cells to neutralize and protect against free radicals. Working in tandem with antioxidant nutrients supplied by our diet, such as vitamin A, carotenes, vitamin C, vitamin E, copper, manganese, selenium, and zinc, these enzymes maintain healthy cell function in a variety of ways. As a result, so long as there is an adequate supply of oxygen, water, antioxidant nutrients, and enzymes in the body, cell damage is kept to a minimum. But when our bodies become deficient in any one of these health-enhancing agents, the cells are overrun by free radicals and the antioxidant defenses become unable to maintain their protective shield. This occurs whenever the body's production of antioxidant enzymes and our intake of antioxidant nutrients fall below what is needed to maintain good health. Poor diet, physical and emotional stress, exposure to pollutants, and lack of sleep all contribute to this decline in enzyme production. Escaping such stressors altogether is practically impossible in today's fast-paced world, but help is available in the form of vitamins and other nutritional antioxidant supplements that can offer substantial help in preventing disease and maintaining proper immune function.

The following table contains recommended dosages for the most common antioxidant vitamins and minerals, all of which should be part of anyone's daily regimen for creating and maintaining optimal health. *Please note that many of the general recommendations below are already included in the Headache Survival regimen as presented above.* There are a number of multivitamin formulas on the market that contain the ingredients listed below, or you can take them separately. Use the higher dosages whenever you are experiencing a headache, exposed to higher levels of stress, diminished sleep, increased exposure to headache triggers, pollutants, and other sources of toxicity, or when you are not eating as well as you should be. Otherwise take at least the minimum dose every day, preferably with your meals.

Table 4.4

Recommended Daily Nutritional Supplements

Vitamin C (as polyascorbate or ester C)—1,000 to 2,000 mg 3 times/day

Beta-carotene—25,000 IU 1 or 2 times/day

Vitamin E—400 IU 1 or 2 times/day

B-complex vitamins—50 to 100 mg of each B vitamin per day

Selenium—100 to 200 mcg per day

Zinc arginate—20 to 40 mg per day

Calcium apatite or citrate—1,000 mg per day

Magnesium glycinate—500 mg per day

Chromium polynicotinate (ChromeMate®)—200 mcg per day

Manganese—10 to 15 mg per day

Copper—2 mg per day

In addition to the above, supplementing with **grape seed extract** (100 mg 1 to 2 times/day between meals) is also advisable. The antioxidant properties of this supplement have been found to be 20 times greater than vitamin C and 50 times greater than vitamin E.

Daily supplementation of **flaxseed oil, evening primrose oil,** or other sources of essential fatty acids are recommended as well, especially for treating headaches (see above).

Professional Care Therapies

Headache Survival is a book and a holistic treatment program with a self-care orientation. However, there are instances in which therapies administered by a physician, conventional or holistic, are needed. These situations might include an acute headache that has not improved with self-medication; headaches that are increasing in frequency, duration, and intensity; or headaches that have not responded very well to any of the suggested therapies listed above. It is also perfectly acceptable and not uncommon for an individual with headaches to choose to enhance the results of the Headache Survival Program with a complementary therapy administered by a physician or health care practitioner. The discipline of holistic medicine facilitates self-care while also including the prudent use of both conventional medicine and professional care alternatives, such as *ayurveda, acupuncture, behavioral medicine, Chinese medicine, chiropractic, energy medicine, environmental medicine, homeopathy, naturopathic medicine, nutritional medicine,* and *osteopathic medicine.* Each of these practices offers treatment options for headache. Nutritional and environmental medicine have been presented earlier in this chapter, while behavioral medicine is the subject of the next chapter.

TRADITIONAL CHINESE MEDICINE

Acupuncture has been used for hundreds of years to treat migraine. It is also helpful for tension headache, both acute and chronic-recurrent, and has been effectively used for prevention. About 70 percent of humans and animals respond to acupuncture treatment. People with chronic headaches who did not respond to acupuncture were found to have low endorphin levels. Although it is difficult to study acupuncture in a placebo-controlled manner, studies suggest that it is quite effective in treating the more severe cases of migraine. In one study, 40 percent of patients achieved a 50 to 100 percent reduction in severity and frequency of migraine episodes. In practice, when performed by an O.M.D. (Doctor of Oriental Medicine), acupuncture is usually combined with **Chinese herbal treatment.** To obtain the appropriate herbs, it is essential to diagnose each patient within the context of traditional Chinese medicine (TCM). But even without the use of herbs, acupuncture is still widely regarded as the *most effective alternative approach to the treatment of migraines.* It can be used during a migraine attack for pain relief, but it works better as prevention for recurrent attacks.

Acupuncture sessions are typically spaced twice a week at first and then gradually tapered. In patients with chronic headaches, treatment usually involves ten or more 20-minute sessions. For migraine headaches that cycle with the menstrual period, treatment will need to be continued at a weekly or twice-weekly rate through at least three menstrual cycles. Other types of migraine may require a greater or lesser length of treatment, depending on the specifics of each case.

Traditional Chinese medicine is based on a history, philosophy, and sociology very different from those of the West. Over thousands of years it has developed a unique understanding of how the body works. Practitioners of Chinese medicine see disease as an imbalance between the body's nutritive substances, called yin, and the functional activity of the body, called yang. This imbalance causes a disruption of the flow of vital energy that circulates through pathways in the body known as meridians. This vital energy, called *qi* or *chi* (pronounced "chee"), keeps the blood circulating, warms the body, and fights disease. The intimate connection between the organ systems of the body and the meridians enables the practice of acupuncture to intercede and rebalance the body's energy through stimulation of specific points along the meridians.

People who have used Chinese medicine for a particular physical symptom frequently experience improvement in seemingly unrelated problems. This occurs because the Chinese approach tends to restore the body to a greater degree of balance, thereby enhancing its capacity for self-healing. The entire person is treated, not just the symptom, and the relationship of body, mind, emotions, spirit, and environment are all taken into account.

The World Health Organization has published a list of more than fifty diseases successfully treated with acupuncture. Included on the list are headaches (including migraine), sinusitis, asthma, arthritis, the common cold, constipation, diarrhea, sciatica, and lower-back pain. Acupuncture has also been effective in the treatment of allergies, addictions, insomnia, stress, depression, infertility, and menstrual problems.

Acupressure works according to the same principle as acupuncture, using the same points on the meridians, but with direct finger pressure used in place of needles to stimulate these points. Of the two techniques, acupuncture is generally more effective, but acupressure allows you to do it yourself. Finger acupressure is applied with the flat parts of your fingers, not the tips, and should always be steady and firm, with about 7 pounds of force. Apply pressure for 20 seconds to 1 minute; press the other side if applicable. To learn more about the technique of acupressure, I recommend the book *Acupressure for Everyone,* by Cathryn Bauer. Commonly used acupressure points for headache include:

- Large intestine 4 (Li 4-hoku, or G-Jo #13)—located in the soft tissue between the thumb and index finger, this point is effective for almost any type of headache; see Figure 4-5. To stimulate this point, using your thumb and index finger of your left hand, press the area located in the fleshy web between your thumb and index finger on the backside of your right hand. Experiment with it until you find the tender spot, and, once there, hold it firmly down toward the bone, pressing as deeply as is comfortable. Do this for 20 seconds to a minute and reverse hands. As you do this, you should feel some warmth or a slight flush of perspiration across your forehead, neck, or shoulders. Most people find that they feel immediately relaxed, and others say this point "erases" their headache.
- Bladder 2 (B 2)—these two points are located below the inner aspect of the eyebrow, in the upper hollows of the eye socket, where the eyebrow meets the bridge of the nose; good for frontal headaches, vascular, tension, eyestrain, and sinus conditions; see Figure 4-6.
- Governing Vessel 24.5 (GV 24.5, Yin Tang or "third eye")— located midway between the eyebrows; good for frontal headaches; see Figure 4-6.
- Gallbladder 20 (GB 20)—located at the occipital ridge bilaterally. This point is good for vascular or tension headache on

the sides or the back of the head, especially when associated with digestive upset, vomiting, dizziness, tooth pain, stiff neck, irritability, and neuromotor coordination problems; see Figure 4-7.

- Bladder 60 (B 60)—located in the hollow behind the bony bump of the ankle. Good for pain at the back of the head, neck, or base of the skull, and for lower-back pain; see Figure 4-8.

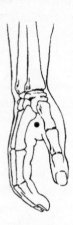

FIGURE 4-5
Li 4-hoku

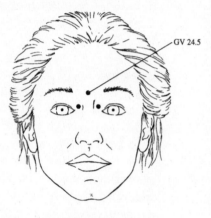

FIGURE 4-6
B 2 and GV 24.5

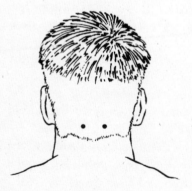

FIGURE 4-7
GB 20

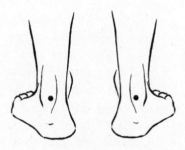

FIGURE 4-8
B 60

ENERGY MEDICINE

Energy medicine modalities such **healing touch, therapeutic touch,** and **Reiki,** can be highly effective for both migraine and tension headache. I have personally seen and performed each of these therapies and have frankly been amazed at the speed with which they can relieve acute headache, both migraine and tension. One study has shown that **transcutaneous electrical nerve stimulation (TENS)** treatment can be successful in treating migraine.

Energy medicine includes a wide range of subtle bioenergetic techniques and the use of both conventional and experimental microcurrent and magnetic energy devices. Energy medicine may well become one of the most important aspects of holistic medicine in the twenty-first century, due to its ability to diagnose and treat disease in the human bioenergy field, often before it manifests physically in the body. Bioenergetic therapies within the field of energy medicine include Therapeutic Touch, Healing touch, Reiki, and jin shin jyutsu. Distance healing, prayer, and meditation are other aspects of energy medicine, as are light, color, sound, and music therapies. Magnetic therapy, t'ai chi, and qigong, and microcurrent therapies (using devices such as the Acuscope and cranial electrical stimulation tools, such as TENS) also fall under the heading of energy medicine. Most of these therapies have the potential to improve the flow of blood and life-force energy (qi, prana, or bioenergy) to the brain and muscles of the scalp, neck, and shoulders. In the hands of a skilled practitioner nearly all of these therapies can benefit headache.

MANUAL MEDICINE

Manual therapies such as **massage** (especially **neuromuscular therapy** for trigger points), **osteopathy** (especially **craniosacral** therapy), **reflexology,** and **chiropractic** are all potentially effective for tension headache, as well as in those cases of migraine in which muscle tension is a trigger. Research has shown massage to be helpful for chronic tension headaches, and as an adjunctive treatment for migraine. The results of studies on chiropractic treatment for tension headache are mixed, while one study evaluating chiropractic treatment for migraine revealed comparable results to medication. Each of these modalities is best performed by a well-trained practitioner.

Osteopathic Medicine

As an osteopathic physician, the art and science of healing with which I'm most familiar is osteopathic medicine, which is essentially *holistic* medicine. It was founded and developed by Andrew Taylor Still, M.D., in 1874. D.O. stands for Doctor of Osteopathic medicine, and D.O.s are fully licensed physicians with unlimited rights and privileges to practice in all fifty states in the United States. D.O.s who have graduated from an osteopathic medical school have completed at a minimum a four-year undergraduate degree, four years of osteopathic medical education at one of the nineteen accredited osteopathic medical schools, and several years of residency training depending on their specialty and area of expertise. D.O.s practice in all medical and surgical specialties, with the greatest percentage of practitioners being in primary care—family practice, pediatrics, and internal medicine.

A. T. Still was a fourth-generation M.D. who, after losing three of his own children one winter to an epidemic of meningitis, began to question the completeness of his medical training. He also suffered from terrible headaches for which he had found no solution in the medical model of his day. In the truly Hippocratic tradition, he became a seeker of answers to his own challenging medical problem. After healing his own headaches, he became widely known for his effective, non-invasive, hands-on approach, and was referred to as a "bone-setter." Dr. Still was unsuccessful in his attempts to have his ideas and methods incorporated into the traditional medical model. Since his apprentices (seven-year apprenticeships were the accepted method of medical training in his day) were being taught medical "heresy," they were not granted the traditional M.D. degree. Instead, they were called D.O.s—Doctors of Osteopathy. (The Latin root *osteo* means "bone," and *patheia* is Greek for "passion" or "suffering.")

When medical schools opened around the turn of the twentieth century, osteopathic students were still thought to be medical heretics, and thus began the two different forms of complete medical training, with two separate medical degrees—M.D. and D.O. Today, osteopathic medical schools have a four-year curriculum very similar to those of allopathic schools, with most of the same courses and textbooks but with several profound differences. Osteopathic medicine has at its core a holistic philosophy and highly developed system of manual diagnostics and treatment techniques that are designed to stimulate our own innate healing and homeostatic mechanisms. The holistic principles upon which osteopathic medicine was founded are as follows:

1. *A person is a complete dynamic unit of function composed of body, mind, and spirit.* Osteopathic medicine recognizes the importance and uniqueness of each of these three elements in every individual and their relationship to disease and optimal health.
2. *The body possesses self-regulatory mechanisms that are self-healing in nature.* The primary objective of the osteopathic physician is to remove the obstacles to health, thereby enabling the body to seek its own path back toward health.
3. *Structure and function are interrelated at all levels.* Therefore, if there is an asymmetry, restriction of motion, or tissue texture change present (these are called *somatic dysfunctions* by osteopathic physicians), one can predict a subsequent alteration in function of the same or referred regions.
4. *Rational treatment is based on understanding and integrating the previous three principles.* Osteopathic medicine, in fact, offers a unique way of looking at a patient and their disease. It is based on a **whole person** perspective, an awareness that the body can heal itself and that its natural state is one of **optimal health,** combined with a scientific focus on understanding and treating the **causes** of disease.

Osteopathic manipulative treatment is as much an art as it is a science, and therefore each patient with headaches may be treated a bit differently by an osteopathic physician. A thorough osteopathic structural exam from foot to head should precede any assumptions that all headaches have their origins in the head and neck. This means that because of the interconnectedness of the body, the aching head could possibly manifest symptoms as a result of compensating for a primary structural problem elsewhere in the body that might be obstructing the flow of blood and nutrients into the head. If other primary problem sites are not ruled out and/or diagnosed and treated appropriately, the headache could be treated repeatedly without significant improvement. This is often the case when one forgets that the body is a complete unit. Attempting to segment it often results in inadequate or unsuccessful treatment.

Osteopathic Manipulative Treatment (OMT) is often highly effective for headaches of various types, especially those related to excess or imbalanced tension. OMT helps patients suffering from headaches, which are really just the result of underlying imbalances or disturbances, by addressing the observable, palpable changes that are present; these areas of change are said to have *somatic dysfunction*. And simply stated, somatic dysfunction is considered to be present whenever there is asymmetry, alterations in normal range of motion, and tissue texture changes. By addressing these areas of somatic dysfunction with OMT, there are many neurophysiologic changes that occur, favoring overall health and decreasing headache intensity, duration, and frequency. The positive neurophysiologic changes that occur generally promote improved muscle tension and subsequent joint balance, improved local as well as overall flexibility, decreased pain, and normalized circulation.

Research that has been done in the past on patients with headaches and migraines as well as in studies that are currently being conducted, look to see if there are any particular OMT technique styles or approaches that are superior to others. The clinical results support the use of many different types of OMT techniques and approaches, with the most commonly reported as follows:

1. Cranial osteopathy—also known as *osteopathy in the cranial field* or *craniosacral therapy,* this is a system of diagnosis and treatment originally described and developed by William Garner Sutherland, D.O. He graduated from the American School of Osteopathy in 1900 and worked on developing what would become cranial osteopathy over the next fifty-plus years. His first publication on this subject, called the *Cranial Bowl,* was published in 1939. The underlying principles behind cranial osteopathy are the following:

   a. There is an inherent motion of the brain and spinal cord.
   b. There is regular fluctuation of the cerebrospinal fluid.
   c. There is inherent mobility of the intracranial and intraspinal membranes.
   d. There is articular mobility of the cranial bones.
   e. There is involuntary mobility of the sacrum between the hipbones.

   A practitioner of cranial osteopathy evaluates and treats the entire body of the patient but is particularly good at diagnosing and addressing structural alterations in the head and sacrum (bone at the base of the spine). This can be of significant benefit to a headache or migraine sufferer with a structural or neurophysiologic problem contributing to their pain. Cranial technique is usually gentle and rarely induces pain. There are intra-oral (fingers in your mouth) techniques as well as techniques that are performed on the outside of the head. The sacrum will be checked as well due to the strong connection between the sacrum and the skull via the dura mater (literally translated, this means "hard mother"), which acts as a protective sheath covering the brain and spinal cord. Cranial manipulation can improve the way the body functions by eliminating obstruction, inflammation, and infection. Another very important benefit associated with cranial manipulation is that it tends to normalize autonomic nervous system imbalances. The autonomic nervous system is that part of the nervous system that controls "automatic" actions in the body, such as heart rate and breathing. It has been divided into a sympathetic and parasympathetic component—the sympathetic being associated with "fight-or-flight" stress responses, the parasympathetic with relaxation responses. Autonomic nervous system imbalances have been linked with many diseases, allergic hyperreactivity, and widespread effects influencing all parts and actions of the body. Thus, cranial osteopathy can be an extremely effective modality for treating a person with headaches and migraines, as well as many other disease conditions.

2. Soft Tissue and Myofascial Release (ST/MFR)—involves gentle and sometimes not-so-gentle manipulation of the muscles and the fascia that surround them, to promote balance and normalization of somatic dysfunction. These techniques promote ease of movement, decreased muscle tension, and normalization of circulation. As these changes often significantly improve posture, which in many individuals contributes greatly to the development of their headaches, it is often a highly effective approach for someone suffering from headaches and migraines.

3. Counterstrain, Facilitated Positional Release and Ligamentous Articular Release (CoS/FPR/LAR)—all involve a gentle balancing of the muscles and ligaments supporting and influencing specific regions of the body. These techniques are extremely useful in particularly tender and painful areas and are generally well tolerated when other techniques are not. When successfully performed, they result in marked pain relief and improvement in motion, which in turn promote normalization of circulation, and often result in the successful treatment of the patient's headache or migraine.

4. Muscle Energy Technique (MET)—involves using the patient's own muscular efforts in correcting areas of somatic dysfunction. Generally, the physician will take the patient's body region to a point where it will not comfortably move (barrier) and ask the patient either to try to move the body region back the way it came from or more into the direction the doctor was moving it. In either case, the physician will not permit any motion by applying an isometric resistance against the patient's efforts. After a few seconds of effort the patient will be instructed to relax and the physician will proceed to move the restricted body region farther in the direction that it previously would not comfortably go. This may be performed several times or until the motion and overall tone of the region have improved. When this is successfully performed it often will result in improvement of the patient's headache or migraine.

5. High Velocity Low Amplitude (HVLA)—involves a rapid thrust through a very small range of motion. This is useful when there is a "locking" or decreased movement of a joint, since it helps to increase free motion and often will result in immediate pain relief. In patients suffering from headaches or migraines, these areas of somatic dysfunction are often found in the upper thoracic and cervical regions (upper back and neck). When these areas are successfully mobilized (treated), the result is often improvement of headache and migraine symptoms. Please note that care must be taken to not overuse this particular technique style because it can potentially lead to hypermobility and joint laxity, thus potentially aggravating symptoms and causing inflammation.

6. Low Velocity High Amplitude (LVHA)—involves gently and slowly moving a patient's body regions through as full a range of motion as possible. This encourages normalization of joint motion and muscle tension, promotes release of synovial fluid (enhancing joint nourishment and lubrication), and promotes normalization of circulation. It is often an excellent way to help restore motion and lengthen

muscles that have been chronically shortened due to poor posture or pain, and thus can significantly help a patient with headaches or migraines.

As you've read in this chapter, headaches are a complex problem with multiple contributing factors requiring a comprehensive holistic approach to effectively treat them. OMT is nearly always successful in allowing the patient greater overall function and a reduction in pain. This often helps people with headaches develop a means to improve their posture and overall fitness levels, diminish use of medications, miss less work and other activities, and learn to be in better communication with their body. It can be a valuable addition to the Headache Survival Program.

Chiropractic (Greek for "done by hand") was developed more than one hundred years ago by David Daniel Palmer, with the primary goal of maintaining the health of the nervous system through the adjustment of bones and joints. Chiropractic theory holds that spinal misalignment (called subluxation) interferes with the flow of vital energy, or what Palmer described as the body's "innate intelligence." Since the nervous system's primary pathway is along the spine, when any part of the spine is subluxated, nerve impulses can be impeded and eventually result in dis-ease in the body's various organs. Chiropractors (or D.C.s) restore spinal alignment with a variety of adjustment and manipulation techniques and comprise a large portion of the alternative practitioners in the United States. Many chiropractors also use kinesiology (muscle testing) and provide nutritional counseling in their practices. Chiropractic can be very helpful in treating headache, especially when the pain has resulted from misaligned or subluxated vertebra.

Naturopathic detoxification may be useful in treating all headaches, but must be done under the supervision of an experienced naturopathic physician.

Ayurveda, the traditional medicine of India, can be helpful for both migraine and tension headaches when it is practiced by a skilled practitioner. The same is true of ***homeopathy.*** Systematic constitutional homeopathy is required to treat migraine and can only be practiced by a highly trained practitioner. Symptomatic homeopathic treatment for tension headache should also be performed by a trained homeopath but is not as challenging a problem as migraine. For symptomatic treatment of tension headache, the following remedies are often prescribed in 12× to 30C dilution, taken as 3 to 5 pellets every 1 to 4 hours until relief is obtained: aconitum, belladonna, bryonia, gelsemium, arnica, and nux vomica.

4. Exercise and Rest

No discussion of physical health would be complete without including the subject of exercise and physical activity. Regular exercise has the potential to contribute more to the condition of optimal health than any other health practice. Yet, in spite of exercise's many proven benefits, we are becoming an increasingly sedentary nation. This is especially true of our children, who are becoming fatter (25 percent are overweight), weaker, and slower than ever before.

Numerous studies show that sedentary people, on average, don't live as long or enjoy as good health as those who get regular aerobic exercise in the form of brisk walking, running, swimming, cycling, rebounding, or similar workouts. In fact, some researchers now believe that lack of exercise may be a more significant risk factor for decreased life expectancy than the *combined* risks of cigarette smoking, high cholesterol, being overweight, and high blood pressure. Simply put, *being unfit means being unhealthy.*

The benefits of regular exercise and physical activity include **lessening of tension (and tension headaches);** *decreased* "fight-or-flight" response, depression, anxiety, smoking, drug use, and incidence of heart disease and cancer; *increased* self-esteem, positive attitudes, joy, spontaneity, mental acuity, mental function, aerobic capacity, and enhanced energy; *increased* muscular strength and flexibility; and *improved* quality of sleep. Regular exercise also results in an increased muscle-to-fat ratio and increased longevity (people who are least fit have a mortality rate three and a half times that of those who are most fit).

Some of the more pronounced benefits of regular exercise occur with older women. A seven-year study conducted by the University of Minnesota School of Public Health tracked the physical activity levels of over 40,000 women, all of whom were postmenopausal and ranged in age from fifty-five to sixty-nine. The results showed that women who exercised at least four times a week at high intensity had up to a 30-percent lowered risk of early death compared to women in the same age group who were sedentary. But even infrequent exercisers among participants in the study (once per week) experienced reduced mortality rates.

In selecting an exercise program, choose a blend of activities that will increase *aerobic capacity, strength,* and *flexibility.* A regimen focused solely on strength conditioning, such as weight lifting, while providing strength, does little to increase aerobic capacity and can even diminish flexibility. Adding a stretching routine and an aerobic workout on alternate days will provide a much more effective exercise practice.

Aerobic Exercise

The word *aerobic* means "with oxygen." Aerobic exercise refers to prolonged exercise that requires extra oxygen to supply energy to the muscles. In general, aerobic activities cause moderate shortness of breath, perspiring, and doubling of the resting pulse rate. A few words of conversation should be possible at the height of activity; otherwise the workout may in fact be too strenuous. One study, published in 1992 in the journal *Headache,* found aerobic exercise to release tension and diminish the frequency and intensity of migraine episodes. Aerobic exercise is, in fact, an essential part of the holistic treatment for headache. Important aspects of this program should include a gradual warm-up and cool-down and avoidance of overheating, excessive sun exposure, and dehydration.

Aerobic exercise is based on maintaining your *target heart rate,* producing greater benefits to the cardiovascular system, and providing more oxygen to the body than any other form of exercise. To determine what your target heart rate should be, use the following formula: 220 minus your age, multiplied by 60 to 85 percent. Keep in mind that 60 percent is considered low-intensity aerobic exercise, with 70 percent being moderate and 85 percent being high intensity. For example, a forty-year-old's target heart rate is between 108 and 153 beats per minute. To accurately determine your pulse, use your index and middle finger to feel the pulse on the thumb side of your wrist or at your neck, just below the jaw. Using a watch with a second hand, count the number of beats in 60 seconds, which will give you your heart rate in beats per minute (or count for 15 seconds and multiply by 4).

When you have attained your target heart rate—for the average person that should take about five to ten minutes of exercising—try to maintain it for at least twenty minutes. It is also beneficial to cool down by working out at a slower heart rate and with less intensity for an additional five to ten minutes before you end your session.

The most convenient forms of aerobic exercise involving the least amount of wear and tear on the body are brisk walking, hiking, swimming, rebounding (jumping on a mini-trampoline), and cycling. Cross-country skiing, if convenient, can also provide a very good aerobic workout. Jogging can also be effective, but to avoid injury, it is recommended that you stretch thoroughly before and after each run, use good running shoes and orthotics—if indicated—and supplement with vitamin C, calcium, and collagen to strengthen your bones, cartilage, muscles, and tendons. Treadmills, rowing machines, stair climbers, stationary bikes, and cross-country ski machines also offer an opportunity for excellent indoor aerobics, as do low-impact aerobics classes. Racquetball, handball, badminton, singles tennis, and basketball provide good aerobic workouts as well.

The keys to a successful aerobic routine are consistency and comfort. Aerobic conditioning does not have to entail a great deal of time, nor does it have to be painful. Find an activity that you can enjoy and keep it fun. Remember, too, that low to moderate aerobic exercise for 45 minutes is just as beneficial as high intensity for 20 minutes. *Do not begin any aerobic activity in the heat of an emotional crisis, especially intense anger.* Wait at least 15 to 20 minutes to avoid the risk of heart attack or arrhythmias that can be triggered under such circumstances. In addition, make sure your aerobic exercise precedes meals by at least half an hour, or follows them by at least two and a half hours, in order to avoid indigestion.

Exercise outdoors if you live or work where it is convenient and safe to do so (specifically with regard to automobile traffic and outdoor air quality and temperature). When you exercise, you may increase your intake of air by as much as ten times your level at rest. The combination of fresh air and sunshine provides greater health benefits than indoor exercise. For migraineurs and chronic respiratory disease sufferers (sinusitis and asthma especially), and for those practicing respiratory preventive medicine, air quality is a critical factor in determining where and when to exercise. Ozone, possibly the most harmful air pollutant, is created by the combination of nitrogen oxides, hydrocarbons, and sunlight. A bright sunny day in the downtown area of most large cities will produce high concentrations of ozone. The EPA considers air unhealthy when ozone levels top 0.125 parts per million. However, in a study conducted by New York University's Morton Lippman, M.D., thirty healthy adults showed decreases in lung capacity during a half-hour of exercise at ozone levels below the federal limit.

If you know that air pollution is a headache trigger, then I suggest scheduling exercise around the rise and fall of pollution levels. In the summer, ozone builds up during the morning, reaches its maximum late in the afternoon, and then ebbs in the evening. In the winter, ozone isn't such a problem, but cold night air can trap a layer of carbon monoxide, nitrogen dioxide, sulfur dioxide, and particulates that can linger into the early morning. A good general practice is to do outdoor exercise in the morning during the summer and in the evening during the winter. However, if ozone levels are generally high, someone with migraine would probably do better exercising indoors.

If you are used to walking, biking, or jogging along main

roads, lung specialists recommend that you stay away from these high-traffic areas during rush hour. Avoid waiting beside stop signs or stoplights, where carbon monoxide builds up. Henry Going, M.D., a UCLA pulmonologist, says, "I've seen guys jogging in place next to cars at stoplights. You might as well smoke a cigarette." On windy days, pollution disperses quickly as you move away from the road. On calm days, it can extend about sixty feet from either side of the road.

If all of these concerns pose too great an obstacle, if you live in a highly polluted city, or if you experience a headache, wheeze, cough, or tightness in your chest during your workout, it's time to head indoors for aerobic exercise. Remember that mouth breathing during exercise bypasses the nose and sinuses, your body's natural air filter, so try to remember to *breathe through your nose*. Ozone levels in most homes, gyms, and pools are about half that of the outdoors—even less with a good air-conditioning system.

Moderate exercise is less strenuous than aerobic, but it is still beneficial. In a research project at the University of Minnesota School of Public Health, moderate exercise was defined as rapid walking, bowling, gardening, yard work, home repairs, dancing, and home exercise, conducted for about an hour daily. A treadmill test determined that those who got this much leisure-time exercise had healthier hearts than those who got less or none. There was no added benefit in doing more than an hour's worth of physical activity. Robert E. Thayer, Ph.D., a professor of psychology at California State University, Long Beach, has found that brisk walks only ten minutes long can increase people's feelings of energy (sometimes for several hours), reduce tension, and make personal problems appear less serious. Not only does it nourish mind and body, *walking is also by far the easiest, safest, and least expensive (you need only comfortable shoes) form of exercise.* Briskly walking two miles at 3.5 to 4 miles per hour (or 17- to 15-minute miles) burns nearly as many calories as running at a moderate pace, and confers similar fitness benefits. By swinging your arms, you'll burn 5 to 10 percent more calories and get an upper-body workout as well.

Strength Conditioning

Building and maintaining muscle strength is another essential component of your overall exercise program. Strength conditioning falls under the following three categories: *Strengthening without aids* includes calisthenics such as sit-ups, push-ups, jumping jacks, and swimming. *Strengthening with aids* includes chin-ups, dips, weight lifting, and training on weight machines. And *strengthening with aerobics* involves various forms of interval training that can be done running, bicycling, jumping rope, circuit training with weight machines, and working out on a heavy bag. The goal of interval training is to work intensively, reaching your maximum heart level for a short interval, then lowering the level of activity to recover. Repeating this process while maintaining your heart rate in its target zone reduces recovery time, strengthens various muscle groups, and conditions the cardiovascular system.

Weight training is perhaps the most popular form of strength-conditioning exercise. To design a weight program to meet your specific needs, consult with a personal trainer, who will most likely advise you to work out two or three times a week. It isn't necessary to lift a lot of weight to build and tone muscle. If muscle tone and definition is your goal, best results will be achieved using less weight and more repetitions. To build mass, increase the amount of weight you use and do fewer repetitions. Remember to breathe *out* (especially important for asthmatics, and be sure NOT to hold your breath during weight training) as you exert effort, and for free-weight exercises it is advisable to work with a spotter. Also, wear a weight belt to help keep your spine properly aligned. If you are unable to work with a personal trainer, refer to the list of recommended books for helpful guidelines in designing your strength-conditioning program.

Increasing Flexibility

The final component of a good exercise program addresses flexibility. This includes stretching exercises, yoga, and tai chi. Exercise that promotes flexibility also significantly contributes to strength and function by allowing the body's muscle groups to perform at maximum efficiency. Lack of flexibility can severely inhibit physical performance, increase the potential for injury, and compromise posture. Muscles exist in a state of static tension wherein contrasting sets of muscles exert similar force to create a state of balance. When muscles become weak or inflexible, this balance is disrupted, resulting in reduced function or postural misalignment. Additional benefits of muscle flexibility include improved circulation, enhanced suppleness of connective tissue (tendons and ligaments), decreased risk of injury, and greater body awareness.

Stretching exercises

Some form of stretching is recommended before and after both aerobic and strengthening workouts. Before you begin stretching, do five minutes of movement to warm up your muscles and body core. This will enhance your circulation and make stretching easier. Never stretch to the point of pain. Ideally, you should feel a tension in the affected muscle or muscle group that you are working. As you do, breathe into the stretch to elongate and relax the muscle group as you hold the posture for 20 to 30 seconds. Repeat each stretch at least twice. You should notice that your range increases on the second and third repetitions. A few minutes of daily stretching will noticeably improve your well-being over time.

Stretching is particularly helpful for most people with tension headaches. Their chronic headache pain may lead to pain in the neck, spine, muscles, and joints, and is often associated with poor posture while sitting or standing. Stretching and strengthening exercises can help decrease pain and enhance mobility. These exercises can be learned from a physical therapist and should be practiced regularly.

Yoga

Yoga, a Sanskrit word meaning "to yoke," refers to a balanced practice of physical exercise, breathing, and meditation to unify body, mind, and spirit, making yoga one of the most effective and ancient forms of holistic self-care. The benefits of this five-thousand-year-old system of mind/body training to improve flexibility, strength, and concentration are well documented. The basis of yoga is the *breath,* a variant of abdominal or belly breathing called *oujai* breathing. There are a number of yogic systems; *hatha yoga* is most well-known in the West. Hatha yoga postures, or *asanas,* affect specific muscle groups and organs to impart physical strength and flexibility, as well as emotional and mental peace of mind.

There are a variety of hatha yoga forms available. Initially it is a good idea to receive instruction for at least a few months, due to the subtleties involved in yoga practice that are not apparent without firsthand experience of its practice under the guidance of a qualified yoga instructor. Although I'm not aware of any studies on the therapeutic benefits of yoga for headache, the relaxation and tension release resulting from the regular practice of yoga could contribute significantly to the prevention of both tension and migraine headache.

Tai chi

Sometimes referred to as *meditation in motion,* tai chi or tai chi chuan, like yoga, is thousands of years old. It involves slow-motion movements integrated with focused belly breathing and visualization and is practiced daily by tens of millions of people in mainland China. The goal of tai chi is to move *qi* ("chee"), or *vital life-force energy,* along the various meridians, or energetic pathways, of the body's various organ systems. According to traditional Chinese medicine, when the flow of *qi* is balanced and unobstructed, both blood and lymph flow are enhanced and the body's neurological impulses function at optimal capacity. The result is greater vitality, resistance to disease, better balance, stimulation of the "relaxation response," increased oxygenation of the blood, deeper sleep, and increased body/mind awareness. Like yoga, the regular practice of tai chi could be quite beneficial for preventing both migraine and tension headache. Although not as well known as yoga in this country, tai chi is rapidly gaining in popularity, and tai chi instructors can be found in most metropolitan areas. After being taught the basic movements of tai chi, you can practice them almost anywhere to instill a centeredness and sense of calm and to alleviate stress.

Aerobic exercise was an integral part of the program I used to cure my own chronic sinusitis, and it is still the most enjoyable part of my daily routine. If you're just beginning a regular exercise program, it won't take long before you start looking forward to your exercise session as one of the highlights of your day. The benefits that you will soon realize will help to increase your motivation to continue. You may eventually do it every day, although research has shown no increased cardiovascular benefits beyond five days a week (three times a week is minimum). However, exercise does much more than merely benefit your heart. As these aerobic workouts strengthen your heart and lungs directly, your ability to provide oxygen to every part of your body is enhanced—and this, after all, is the scientific basis of physical health. It will help you to relax, release tension, oxygenate your brain, and perhaps stabilize serotonin metabolism. Regular aerobic exercise might possibly become the key element in your treatment program to overcome your headache condition.

As a human animal, you can experience many of life's greatest pleasures only through your body. Regular exercise can add immeasurably to your enjoyment of life and heighten your sense of well-being.

Sleep and Relaxation

While diet, the use of supplements, and exercise can all benefit physical health, improve immune function, and reduce inflammation, perhaps the most powerful and overlooked key to overall well-being is sleep. The average person requires between eight and nine hours of uninterrupted sleep, yet in the United States we average between six and eight hours, with an estimated 50 million Americans suffering from insomnia.

Lack of sleep and its resulting depression of the immune system can be a factor in many chronic health conditions. I've seen it repeatedly in patients with headaches. Additional sleep is therefore an essential component in the holistic treatment of this condition. You've already learned in Chapter 2 that irregular sleep patterns, including either lack of sleep or oversleeping, are important migraine triggers. Besides lowered immune function, sleep deprivation can also cause a decrease in productivity, creativity, and job performance and can affect mood and mental alertness. In cases of insomnia, most incidents of sleep deprivation are due to a specific stress-producing event. While stress-induced insomnia is usually temporary, it may persist well beyond the precipitating event to become a chronic problem. Overstimulation of the nervous system (especially from caffeine, salt, or sugar) or simply the fear that you can't fall asleep are other common causes.

Researchers have identified two types of sleep: *heavy* and *light*. During heavier, or nonrapid-eye-movement (NREM) sleep, your body's self-repair and healing mechanisms are revitalized, enabling your body to repair itself. During lighter, rapid-eye-movement (REM) sleep, you dream more, releasing stress and tension. (For more on dreams, see Chapter 5.)

Conventional medicine commonly prescribes sleeping pills for insomnia and other sleep disorders, but as with almost all medications, there are unpleasant side effects to contend with, as well as the risk of developing dependency. A more holistic approach to ensuring adequate sleep begins with establishing a regular bedtime every night so that you can begin to re-attune yourself to nature's rhythms. By not awakening to an alarm clock, you allow your body to get the amount of sleep that it requires. Try going to sleep earlier if you find you still need an alarm clock.

Many insomniacs (those that awaken in the middle of the night and can't fall back to sleep) have developed the habit of "clock watching" during the night when they wake up. They typically have an alarm clock with bright red digits glaring at them in the darkness, and they may have actually trained their unconscious mind to *look for* those preprogrammed times. The silent message that they consistently hear (especially before going to bed) is "I wake up every night at ——— A.M." As this pattern of awakening too early continues, they are literally creating the expectation to awaken at their designated time, and their hormones and nervous system follow their explicit instructions. They can break this habit by not checking the time, turning the clock around so that's it's facing away from them, or turning it off! When they do, most are able to end their insomnia.

According to Ayurvedic medicine (the traditional medicine of India), the circadian rhythm, caused by the earth rotating on its axis every twenty-four hours, has a counterpart in the human body. Modern science has confirmed that many neurological and endocrine functions follow this circadian rhythm, including the sleep-wakefulness cycle. Ayurveda teaches that the ideal bedtime for the deepest sleep and for being in sync with this natural rhythm is 10 P.M. Unfortunately, most people with insomnia dread bedtime and go to bed later, when sleep tends to be somewhat lighter and more active. Ayurveda also states that eight hours of sleep beginning at 9:30 P.M. is twice as restful as eight hours beginning at 2 A.M. It is also important in resetting your biological clock to get up early and at the same time every day, regardless of when you go to bed. Establishing an early wake-up time (6 or 7 A.M.) is essential for overcoming insomnia. You'll eventually begin to feel sleepier earlier in the evening, and even if you aren't actually sleeping by 10 P.M., you'll benefit just by resting in bed at that hour.

Other natural remedies include (several of these were discussed on pages 122–24 as part of the treatment for tension headache):

- vitamin B-complex, 50 to 100 mg daily with meals. The best food sources of the B vitamins are liver, whole grains, wheat germ, tuna, walnuts, peanuts, bananas, sunflower seeds, and blackstrap molasses.
- niacinamide (vitamin B_3) up to one gram (1,000 mg) at bedtime, for people who have trouble staying asleep, not falling asleep
- calcium and magnesium, 500 to 1,000 mg of each within 45 minutes of bedtime

- chamomile, passionflower, hops, skullcap, and especially valerian herbs. They are natural sedatives that do not alter the
  quality of sleep the way prescription and over-the-counter
  drugs do; they can all be taken as a tea, while valerian and
  passionflower are available in stronger dosages in a tincture
  form.
- kava kava is another useful herb for both anxiety and insomnia. Recommended dosage for sleep is two to three capsules
  (60 to 75 mg per capsule) an hour before bedtime.
- tryptophan, three to five grams 45 minutes before retiring,
  and at least one and a half hours after eating protein; adding
  B_6 to the tryptophan along with fruit juice can improve results. Tryptophan is available by prescription only.
- 5-hydroxytrytophan (5-HTP), 100 to 250 mg before bed
- Melatonin, a hormone produced by the pineal gland in response to darkness, is most effective for difficulty falling
  asleep; recommended dosage ranges from 1 to 4 mg, one half
  hour to one hour before bed. Melatonin can also be used for
  sleep maintenance with a sustained-release 1-mg preparation.
- hot bath or hot tub
- breathing exercises and/or meditation to relax muscles and
  relieve tension

Most important, don't worry about lost sleep, since in most
cases anxiety is what caused the problem in the first place. If you
can learn to relax without drugs, you will have cured your sleeping problems while giving your immune system a powerful
boost. Nearly all of the recommendations in Chapters 5 and 6
will help you to achieve this goal.

Relaxation is another essential ability that promotes physical
health. The word is derived from the Latin *relaxare,* meaning "to
loosen." Relaxation is a way to allow the mind to return to a
natural state of equilibrium, creating a state of balance between
the right and left brain. It is also a highly effective means of stress
reduction.

Relaxation is a skill that can be improved upon with practice;
therefore, it is recommended that you take time each day to

relax. This can be achieved as easily as taking a few deep abdominal breaths or simply shifting your focus away from your problems and concerns, or through any activity that engages your creative and physical faculties. Such activities include reading and writing, gardening, taking a walk, painting, singing, playing music, doing crafts, or any other hobby that you enjoy for its own sake, without the need to be concerned about your performance. Committing two to three evening hours a week to the hobby or activity of your choice will help make relaxation a natural and regular part of your daily experience. The ability to relax and shift gears away from the competitive drive that compels most of us in our society holds the key to greater health.

SUMMARY

Obviously the entire physical health component of the Headache Survival Program is too comprehensive for anyone to be expected to follow every one of these recommendations. However, there are many people who have obtained significant relief from their headaches by strictly adhering to just one or two of the components of the Program—the diet, or feverfew and magnesium, or riboflavin and fish oil, and so on. My suggestion to patients is to make a *commitment* to incorporate into your daily life as many of the above recommendations as you are comfortably able to do. Take your time. The more gradual the process, the more likely it is that you'll stay with it. Try adding one new thing each week.

If after three months of consistently adhering (daily practice) to at least three of the above recommendations, you have not yet experienced any change in your symptoms, I would continue with at least the initial breathing/air, water, dietary, feverfew, riboflavin, magnesium, exercise, and sleep recommendations and also consider one of the *professional care therapies*. I would also suggest you begin to add the mental/emotional and spiritual/social aspects (Chapters 5 and 6) of the Headache Survival Program to the holistic approach for treating your headache. Remember, holistic medicine looks at every physical dis-ease as the body's reflection of an imbalance or disharmony in the whole person. *Healing* your headaches entails more than simply modifying your diet or taking an herb or supplement. It might be helpful for you to work with a *holistic physician*. Please refer to the Resource Guide, beginning on page 247, to find one.

However, if you have followed the Headache Survival Program closely for at least three months, you will most likely have noticed a significant improvement. If so, you can begin to gradually reduce the highest dosages of the supplements. There is no hard-and-fast rule for what the new dosages should be. Every individual is somewhat different, and you'll have to find the appropriate level for you. If your symptoms begin to recur, then increase to previous dosages. You can also gradually increase your level of exercise. To maintain and to enhance your improvement, you can also start incorporating more of the *physical* and *environmental health* recommendations for *optimal well-being,* in addition to the suggestions for "Healing the Mind" and "Healing the Spirit" in the next two chapters. Your commitment to these other two components of the Headache Survival Program is essential for *preventing* recurrences and possibly *curing* your headaches.

Committing yourself to a consistent program of eating well, taking the proper supplements, becoming more physically fit, and creating a healthy environment based on the recommendations in this chapter will enable you to achieve improvements in your physical well-being in as little as a few weeks. You may also notice significant improvement in your headache condition. Before long, you will find that your reserves of energy are greater, and that you are physically stronger, more powerful, and more flexible. You will also develop a more positive self-image and feel better about how your body looks and performs in every realm of activity. And if you have been spending more time outdoors, you will feel more connected to and empowered by nature.

Optimal physical health is a feeling of *harmony* within your body. The underlying physical basis will be experienced as an *ef-*

fortless flowing of all bodily functions and fluids. Your breathing will become more abdominal and less restricted, providing a greater supply of oxygen to every cell as it flows through less constricted arteries. Enhanced by an increased intake of water, your circulation will in turn allow your kidneys and bowels more complete elimination of toxins and waste. Your more nutritious diet will provide better nourishment and more energy to your cells. And your more regular and effortless bowel movements will be more conducive to maximum absorption of nutrients. Your body movement and exercise programs will even further facilitate the nourishment of all cells, tissues, and organs.

As you begin to thrive, you will be sleeping more deeply and making time for relaxation. You will enjoy greater sexual energy and often greater endurance and pleasure. You will become more aware and appreciative of the miracle of your own body, and the intelligence and efficiency with which it regulates and heals itself. You will also have a better understanding of how your body relates to and is impacted by the environment surrounding it. You might even develop a sense of how the improved harmony with your environment may enhance your longevity.

Your body is simply working better. As a result, it can provide you with some of life's simplest but greatest pleasures: deep sleep, a pain-free neck and head, uncongested breathing, graceful movement, unrestricted urination, easy bowel movements, enhanced sexual performance, and an awareness of the unimpeded flow of life energy that connects us to one another and to our environment. Such benefits are just the beginning of your journey to optimal well-being. They will continue to become more noticeable as you take more responsibility for your health and follow this chapter's guidelines in the months and years ahead. In the process, you will be creating the foundation necessary for healing the other aspects of holistic medicine's triumvirate—*mind and spirit*—while you are healing your headaches.

Chapter 5

HEALING YOUR MIND
The Mental and Emotional Health Components of the Headache Survival Program

The greatest discovery of any generation is that human beings can alter their lives by altering the attitudes of their minds.

—ALBERT SCHWEITZER

COMPONENTS OF OPTIMAL MENTAL HEALTH

Peace of mind and contentment
- A job that you love doing
- Optimism
- A sense of humor
- Financial well-being
- Living your life vision
- The ability to express your creativity and talents
- The capacity to make healthy decisions

COMPONENTS OF OPTIMAL EMOTIONAL HEALTH

Self-acceptance and high self-esteem
- The capacity to identify, express, experience, and accept all of your feelings, both painful and joyful
- Awareness of the intimate connection between your physical and emotional bodies
- The ability to confront your greatest fears
- The fulfillment of your capacity to play
- Peak experiences on a regular basis

One of the most exciting developments in the field of medicine in recent decades has been the scientific verification that our physical health is directly influenced by our thoughts and emotions. The reverse is also true; overwhelming evidence now exists showing that our physiology has a direct correlation to the ways we habitually think and feel. While Eastern systems of medicine, such as traditional Chinese medicine and Ayurveda, have for centuries recognized these facts and stressed the importance of a harmonious connection between body and mind, in the West this mind–body connection did not begin to be acknowledged until research conducted in the 1970s and '80s conclusively revealed the ability of thoughts, emotions, and attitudes to influence our bodies' immune functions. In fact, many of the scientists exploring this relatively new field of psychoneuroimmunology (PNI) have concluded that *there is no separation between mind and body.*

In order to heal our minds and emotions, it helps to know what we mean by the term *mental health*. From the perspective of holistic medicine, the essence of mental health is peace of mind and feelings of contentment. Being mentally healthy means that you recognize the ways in which your thoughts, beliefs, mental imagery, and attitudes affect your well-being and limit or expand your ability to enjoy your life. It also means knowing that you always have choices about what you think and believe, and are aware of your gifts, are practicing your special talents, working at a job that you enjoy, and being clear about your priorities, values, and goals. People who have made a commitment to their mental health live their lives with rich reserves of humor and optimism. They have chosen a nurturing set of beliefs and attitudes that fill them with peace and hope. Most people who buy this book do so with the belief, however minimal, that they or a loved one will not have to suffer with headaches for the rest of their lives and will free themselves of living with the fear of sudden and incapacitating pain. Since you have read to this point and begun practicing the physical components of the Headache Survival Program, your belief has probably been strengthened considerably. You can determine your own state of mental health by referring to the appropriate section of the Thriving Self-Test at the end of Chapter 3, then use the information in this chapter to improve the areas you may need to work on.

The term *mental health* can be interpreted to include not only our thoughts and beliefs but also our feelings. However, when your focus is specifically on "feelings," this is the realm of *emotional health*. These aspects of ourselves—**mental** and **emotional**—are for the most part inextricably related and together form the **"mind"** aspect of holistic health. As your healing journey progresses, you will increasingly come to recognize how your own distorted or illogical thoughts are the underlying cause of feelings such as anger, depression, anxiety, fear, and unfounded guilt. Learning how to free yourself from such distorted thinking patterns is the goal of this chapter, and of behavioral medicine, the aspect of holistic medicine that deals with this interconnectedness among physical, mental, and emotional health. Behavioral medicine includes professional treatment approaches such as *psychotherapy, mind/body medicine, guided imagery and visualization, biofeedback therapy, hypnotherapy, neurolinguistic programming (NLP), orthomolecular medicine* (the use of nutritional supplements to treat chronic mental disease), *flower essences,* and body-centered therapies like *Rolfing* and *Hellerwork.* However, with the exception of psychotherapy and hypnosis, the focus in this chapter is on proven self-care approaches that you can begin using immediately to heal the mind along with your headaches. They include *creating new beliefs and establishing clear goals, affirmations, breathwork, guided imagery, visualization, meditation, dreamwork, journaling,* and your approaches to both *work* and *play.* Each of these methods can help you become more aware of your habitual thoughts, attitudes, and emotions—both pleasurable and painful—in order to create a mind-set conducive to experiencing optimal health and more effectively meeting your professional goals and personal desires, including freeing yourself from the restraints of disabling headaches.

THE BODY-MIND CONNECTION

Growing numbers of Western scientists and physicians now recognize that *body* and *mind* are not separate aspects of our being, but interrelated expressions of the same experience. Their view is based on the findings of researchers working in the field of *psychoneuroimmunology (PNI)*, also referred to as *neuroscience,* which for the past three decades has shown us that our thoughts, emotions, and attitudes can directly influence immune and hormone function. In light of such research, scientists now commonly speak of the mind's ability to control the body. In large part, this perspective is due to the scientific discovery of "messenger" molecules known as *neuropeptides,* chemicals that communicate our thoughts, emotions, attitudes, and beliefs to every cell in our body. In practical terms, this means that all of us are capable of both weakening or strengthening our immune system according to how we think and feel. Moreover, scientists have also proven that these messages can originate not only in the brain but from every cell in our body. As a result of such studies, scientists now conclude that the immune system actually functions as a "circulating nervous system" that is actively and acutely attuned to our every thought and emotion.

Among the discoveries that have occurred in the field of PNI are the following:

- Feelings of loss and self-rejection can diminish immune function and contribute to a number of chronic disease conditions, including heart attack.
- Feelings of exhilaration and joy produce measurable levels of a neuropeptide identical to interleukin-2, a powerful anti-cancer drug that costs many thousands of dollars per injection.
- Feelings of peace and calm produce a chemical very similar to Valium, a popular tranquilizer.
- Depressive states negatively impact the immune system and increase the likelihood of illness.
- Chronic grief or a sense of loss can increase the likelihood of cancer (and although it has not been scientifically docu-

mented, it is my clinical observation that it increases the likelihood of asthma).

- Anxiety and fear can trigger high blood pressure.
- Feelings of hostility, grief, depression, hopelessness, and isolation greatly increase the risk of heart attack.
- Repressed anger is a factor in many chronic ailments, including sinusitis, bronchitis, headaches, and candidiasis.
- Acknowledgment and expression of feelings strengthen immune responses.
- Anger decreases immunoglobulin A (a protective antibody) in saliva, while caring, compassion, humor, and laughter increase it.
- Chronic stress has a broad suppressive effect on immunity, including the depression of natural killer cells, which attack cancer cells.

As exciting as these discoveries are, the studies that had the greatest impact on me were performed on multiple-personality patients at the National Institutes of Health (NIH). Scientists found that in one personality an individual could have the strongest possible skin reaction to an allergen or be severely nearsighted, but after shifting to another personality (an unconscious process in the *same* body), there was *no skin reaction* to the same allergen and perfectly normal *20/20 vision*! Science is just beginning to understand the depth and power of the connection between mind and body.

The implications of these discoveries are enormous and are producing a paradigmatic shift in physicians' approaches to treating chronic disease. They play an essential role in the Headache Survival Program: If emotions and attitudes can contribute to causing heart disease and cancer, it isn't too difficult to appreciate how they can also play a critical role in causing headaches, both tension and migraine. They are also tremendously empowering for anyone committed to holistic health. Once you accept the fact that there is an ongoing, instant, and intimate communication occurring between your mind and your body via the mechanisms of neuropeptides, you can also see that the person best qualified to direct that communication in your own life is you. Learning how to do so effectively can enable you to become your own twenty-four-hour-a-day healer by becoming more conscious of your thoughts and emotions and managing them better to improve all areas of your health. The first step in this process is acknowledging that you can no longer afford to continue feeding yourself the same limiting messages you most likely have been conditioned to accept since early childhood. Scientists now estimate that the average person has approximately fifty thousand thoughts each day; yet 95 percent of them are the same as the ones he or she had the day before. Typically such thoughts are not only unconscious but often critical and limiting. For example: "I'll never be completely free of these headaches [or any chronic condition]." "I'll always be dependent on these drugs." "I should've done _____ to have prevented this situation." "I can't realize my greatest potential or fully enjoy my life as long as I'm stuck with this miserable _____." When you're hearing messages like these repeated many times during the course of a typical day, it's easy to understand why for most people with a chronic condition like migraine headache, *fear, anger, hopelessness, sadness,* and *depression* may become their predominant feelings. You've just read that these painful emotions can be associated with weakening the immune system while also contributing to a myriad of physical problems. However, *by consciously taking control of your thoughts and recognizing how they govern your behavior, you can dramatically change your life and heal your dis-ease.* You will gain the freedom to think, feel, and believe as you choose, thereby flooding your body's cells with positive, life-affirming messages capable of contributing to your optimal health.

5. Play/Passion/Purpose

The fifth item on my list of the *essential 8 for optimal health* is a mental/emotional (and spiritual/social) health practice focused on living a life filled with passion. This requires a level of self-awareness that will allow you to better understand and appreciate yourself while recognizing:

- your greatest talents and gifts
- what you most enjoy in life—what feels like play to you
- what would give your life greater meaning
- the purpose of your life—what you believe you came here to do

The next step on your path to optimal health is for you to begin creating a life that is more in accord with the responses to these self-posed questions. I've described this condition (holistic health) as the unlimited and unimpeded free flow of life-force energy through your body, mind, and spirit. The remainder of this and the following chapter provide a variety of approaches to enhance this flow of life energy through your mind and spirit. They will provide you with valuable tools for gaining greater peace of mind, self-acceptance, and the self-esteem required to proceed on your healing path and enjoy more play and passion in your life.

PSYCHOTHERAPY

The field of psychotherapy, an outgrowth of the theories and discoveries of Sigmund Freud, continues to evolve more than a hundred years since its inception. In addition to the mental and emotional benefits commonly attributed to psychotherapy, a growing body of research has documented that physical benefits can also occur. For example, in a study conducted at the UCLA School of Medicine by the late Norman Cousins, a group of cancer patients receiving psychotherapy for ninety minutes a week showed dramatic improvement in their immune systems after only six weeks. During that same period the control group of other cancer patients who received no counseling showed no change in immune function whatsoever.

Psychotherapy, by its very nature, is not a self-care protocol but can be extremely valuable for individuals struggling with deep-rooted mental and emotional problems. The most popular forms of psychotherapy are *classical* or *Freudian psychoanalysis, Jungian psychoanalysis, family therapy, cognitive/behavioral therapy, brief/solution-focused therapy,* and *humanistic/existential therapy.* Though they all share the same goal of helping patients achieve mental health, their approaches can vary widely.

If you feel that psychotherapy may help you, you will gain the most benefit by choosing the approach best suited to your specific needs and objectives. In addition, be aware that the work of psychotherapy is increasingly being conducted by non-psychiatrists, including psychologists, social workers, and pastoral counselors. One of the reasons for this, perhaps, lies in the fact that many of today's patients seeing psychiatrists are given a psychiatric diagnosis (depression, manic-depressive, obsessive-compulsive, etc.) and then treated with drugs, such as the anti-depressant Prozac. This trend within psychiatry, a departure from counseling toward greater drug therapy, makes it a less desirable choice for someone interested in a holistic and self-care approach. While psychotherapeutic drugs can be effective at times, especially over the short term, each of the drugs commonly prescribed by psychiatrists has the potential to cause unpleasant side effects. Equally important, by focusing on treating psychological symptoms with drugs, many psychiatrists are depriving their patients of the opportunity to change their attitudes and behavior and to learn how to understand and grow from their emotional pain. Finally, whichever type of psychotherapist you choose, make sure that he or she is someone with whom you are comfortable. Psychotherapy can be effective only in a situation of trust, so you may wish to interview a number of therapists before making your choice.

BELIEFS, ATTITUDES, GOALS, AND AFFIRMATIONS

In his classic treatise *The Science of Mind,* noted spiritual teacher Ernest Holmes wrote: "Health and sickness are largely externalizations of our dominant mental and spiritual states. A normal healthy mind reflects itself in a healthy body, and conversely, an abnormal mental state expresses its corresponding condition in some physical condition." At the time Holmes wrote those words, in the mid-1920s, modern science was far behind him in understanding how *our thoughts directly influence our physical health.* But today a growing body of evidence not only verifies this fact but also indicates that it is our predominant, habitual beliefs that determine the thoughts we primarily think. Socrates stated that the unexamined life was not worth living. Based on today's research in the field of behavioral medicine, we may paraphrase his statement to say, *"The unexamined belief is not worth believing in."* Yet most of us have never taken the time to actually examine the beliefs we hold, and therefore remain unaware of how they may be influencing our well-being.

The importance of beliefs in the overall scheme of human functioning is confirmed by placebo studies. A placebo is a dummy medication or procedure possessing no therapeutic properties that works only because of our belief in it. Detailed analysis of thirteen placebo studies from 1940 to 1979, including 1,200 patients, found an 82 percent improvement resulting from the use of medications or procedures that subsequently proved to be placebos.

Changing your beliefs is essential to your success with the Headache Survival Program. Most people suffering with migraine have been told by their physicians: "You're going to have to learn to live with this problem"; "The only thing that can be done is to take medication—analgesics, Imitrex, or one of the newer triptans—to control the symptoms"; "If you adhere to the established migraine treatment protocol, you may eventually be able to take less medication"; or "There's nothing that can cure your migraine or cluster headaches [or the majority of diseases]." These statements are, however, only beliefs. They are based on the limitations of modern medical science, a highly scientific and technologically advanced approach to the treatment of disease, and they are delivered to the patient by a highly educated individual in a society that defers to expertise. These pronouncements, which are in some cases death sentences, are quickly accepted by most patients and become a part of their own belief system. The vast majority of people with terminal diseases who accept whatever their doctors tell them (these patients are called "compliant") die very close to their predicted life expectancy. By contrast, patients who challenge their physician's "death sentence" tend to survive much longer, and some of them go on to achieve full recoveries. In *Love, Medicine, & Miracles*, Bernie Siegel, M.D., vividly describes how the beliefs and attitudes of many of his cancer patients affected the outcome of their disease.

Most of the beliefs held by Americans have been defined by the standards, or norms, of our society, but how well does the norm fit you, a unique individual? If all of us attempted to conform, the world would be a boring place, devoid of creativity and innovation. We certainly wouldn't be enjoying the ease of living that technology has provided us were it not for the adventurous few who deviated from the conventional belief system.

Unfortunately, in every culture there is great pressure to conform. It isn't easy, to say the least, to hold beliefs that run counter to prevalent attitudes. Society, friends, and family all tell us we have strayed with phrases such as "You should . . . ," "You ought to . . . ," or—if your belief has caused them a lot of discomfort—"You're crazy!" Most of the time we respond to this pressure by giving up our unreasonable, or even outrageous, beliefs. Ultimately almost all of us would prefer to be accepted and loved by others; besides, we tell ourselves, "It wasn't that big a deal anyway."

Your belief system has a profound impact on your life: what you eat and think; how you dress and behave; what you do for a living; whom you choose to marry, befriend, or live with; how you spend your leisure time; what your values and goals are; and how you define health and quality of life. It also determines the nature of the silent messages you give yourself every day. All of us talk to ourselves, and this internal dialog has a great deal to do with our state of mental health. These messages may be generally self-critical ("You stupid . . ." "Why did I say that?" "Why did I do that?" "How could I . . . ?" "I should've [could've] . . ."); limiting ("I'll never be able to . . ."); or accepting and supportive ("Good job!" "That's fine." "I did the best I could."). Almost all of my patients are very hard on themselves. They are self-critical and put themselves under a great deal of unnecessary pressure, while at the same time most are high achievers. As human beings we are imperfect; all of us make mistakes. The way we respond to these failings is what creates more, or lessens, stress in our lives. Our pattern of response is one we probably have been repeating reflexively since childhood.

A very simple yet powerful exercise that can help you become more conscious of your thoughts, beliefs, and emotions is to devote fifteen minutes writing out all that you are thinking during that time. Do this when you are not likely to be disturbed and don't edit anything out. After a few days of practicing this technique, many of your predominant beliefs will have been expressed on paper. Read them over. If they don't feel nurturing, build confidence and self-esteem, or regenerate you, clearly they are not serving you and need to be either eliminated or changed. Pay particular attention to the *shoulds, coulds,* and *nevers.* Before you discard what you write, examine your statements for possible clues to aspects of your life that may require more of your attention. For instance, if one of your statements reads, "I hate going to work," more than likely you may need to change your attitude about your job, or leave it for one that is more fulfilling and better suited to your talents. (If the thought of leaving your job raises the thought "How will I provide for myself and my family?," realize that this in itself can be a limiting thought. Numerous options will become available to you once you liberate yourself from your old assumptions and beliefs.)

Once you have identified beliefs that are holding you back from your goals and desires or negatively impacting your health, the next step is to begin to *reprogram* your mind with thoughts, ideas, and images more aligned to what you want. One of the most effective ways to do this is through the use of **affirmations,** or positive thoughts that you repeat to yourself either verbally or in writing in order to produce a specific outcome. Affirmations are positive statements repeated frequently, always in the present tense, containing only positive words, and serve as a response to an often-heard negative message or as expression of a goal. For example, if some of the previous critical messages sound familiar to you, two affirmations that would help counteract them are "I love and approve of myself" and "I am always doing the best I can." These positive thoughts create images that directly affect the unconscious, shaping patterns of thought to direct behavior. In doing so, they act as powerful tools to unleash and stimulate the healing energy of love present in great abundance within each of us.

The purpose of affirmations is to replace habitual, limiting thought patterns and beliefs with more nurturing images of how you want your life to be. When affirmations are practiced regularly, they have the power to create optimal health by infusing the immune system with the life energy of *hope,* which triggers the activity of neuropeptides in the cells. Affirmations can be used to address virtually all aspects of your life, enhancing self-esteem, improving the quality of relationships, dealing with illness, and launching a more rewarding career.

Because of the simple nature of affirmations, the greatest challenge in using them is to suspend judgment long enough to allow them to produce the results you desire. When people begin repeating affirmations, they usually don't believe what they're saying (that's why they're saying them), although they would like to. Using affirmations is like reprogramming a computer. Your subconscious mind is the computer that has been receiving the same message for years—as the direct result of the thoughts and beliefs you have held for most, if not all, of your life. Now you are going to change the input with new "software."

Most computers have a total capacity for processing information far beyond the ability of the majority of computer operators to access it. Similarly, neuroscientists believe that the average person uses only 5 to 10 percent of his or her total brain capacity. As mentioned earlier, this average person has about fifty thousand thoughts every day, and it is estimated that 95 percent of them are the same ones he or she had the day before. Since your brain is hearing the same "program" repeated over and over again, it's no wonder you are able to realize only a small fraction of your (and your brain's) full potential. *Mental health will help to develop your creativity—you'll be re-creating yourself— while allowing you greater access to the parts of your brain that have been dormant.* It is in that recreational process that you'll find an almost limitless supply of joy and passion, along with some strong doses of pain to keep you on track.

The best time to say your affirmation is immediately following the negative message you repeatedly give yourself. When you're feeling the frustration of suffering with another headache and thinking to yourself, "This will never go away," you can follow that hopeless comment with the affirmation "I am healing my headaches and my head feels light and clear." Positive statements like this while you're in the midst of practicing abdominal breathing exercises, changing your diet, taking the supplements, and the rest of the Headache Survival Program, will not only help to feel a little better, but will also increase your level of hope. And as your headaches diminish in frequency, duration, and/or intensity, you'll believe the affirmation more and more until it is actually true.

After you read "Emotional Causes of Headache" on page 176, think about how the information regarding some of the more common emotional factors might relate to you. At the same time, you should also consider the content of your often-heard silent messages. If you find that one or more of these specific issues applies to you, then I would recommend creating affirmations to help lessen the harmful impact they may be having on your headaches.

There are a variety of ways to use affirmations. Some people find they get their best results by writing each affirmation ten to twenty times a day. Others prefer to say them out loud, or to record them onto a cassette that they can then play to themselves daily. One powerful technique suggested by Louise Hay, author of the best-selling *You Can Heal Your Life*, is to stare into a mirror and make eye contact with your reflection while verbally repeating each affirmation. Hay notes that this experience tends to bring up feelings of discomfort at first, and recommends that you continue the process until such feelings lessen or fade away altogether. You can experiment with these and other methods until you find the one that works best for you. Here are some other guidelines to ensure that you get the best results from your affirmation program:

1. Always state your affirmation in the present tense, and keep it positive. For example, if one of your goals is to be free of job-related stress, the affirmation *I accomplish my daily responsibilities with ease and satisfaction* will produce far more effective results than statements such as *My job no longer makes me stressful.* The reason affirmations work is that the unconscious accepts them as statements of fact, and immediately begins to reorganize your life experience to match what you are telling it. So state *what you desire,* not what you wish to be free from, and write and say your affirmation in the present tense *as if your desire is already accomplished.*

2. Keep your affirmations short and simple, and no longer than two brief sentences.

3. Say or write each affirmation at least ten to twenty times each day.

4. Whenever you experience yourself thinking or hearing a habitual negative message, counteract it by focusing on your affirmation. Over time, you will find that your tendency to give yourself negative messages will diminish.

5. Schedule a time each day to do your affirmations and adhere to it. Doing something regularly at the same time

each day adds to the momentum of what you are trying to achieve and eventually will become a positive, effortless habit.

6. Repeat your affirmations in the first, second, and third person, using your name in each variation. Using affirmations in the first person addresses the mental conditioning you have given yourself, while affirmations in the second and third person helps to release the conditioning you may have been accepting from others. For example, if your name is Tom and one of your goals is to make more money, you might write: *I, Tom, am earning enough money to satisfy all my needs and desires. You, Tom, are earning enough money to satisfy all your needs and desires. He, Tom, is earning enough money to satisfy all his needs and desires.* In each case, write out or repeat the affirmation ten times.

7. Make a commitment to practice your affirmations for at least sixty days or until you begin experiencing the result you desire.

You can use affirmations to help change any belief that doesn't feel good to you, to help you achieve any goal, or to create the life of your dreams. Most of my patients have come in because of one or more chronic physical or mental problems. Their objectives are clear: to stop living with chronic pain, to stop having sinus infections, to get rid of allergies or asthma, to have more energy, to suffer less anxiety, and so forth. After they have begun to see a definite improvement in their physical condition, which is usually after they have been working on the physical and environmental aspects of the specific holistic medical treatment program (Headache, Arthritis, Sinus, or Asthma Survival Program) for one to three months, I recommend that they create a "wish list" in the form of affirmations. The following is a powerful exercise for transforming your life and creating optimal mental health.

• **List your greatest talents and gifts.** You have several. These are things that are most special about you, or that you do better than most other people. Ask yourself, "What do I most appreciate about myself?"

- **Next, list the things you most enjoy**—both activities and states of being; for example, "I really enjoy just being in the mountains, or on a beach." There will be some overlap with your first list. Many of the activities you enjoy doing are the things you're best at. This exercise is especially important for migraineurs, since they often deprive themselves of fun and are not very good self-nurturers.

- **Next, list the things that have the most meaning for you.** This is important, because if your goal doesn't meaningfully encompass more than one area of your life, or have benefit to others in some way, more than likely it is incomplete, and you will lack the passion necessary to commit to it. As you list the meaningful things in your life, you will more easily recognize the talents and activities you enjoy that are most worth your while.

- **Now make a wish list of all your goals or objectives in every realm of your life**—physical/environmental, mental, emotional, social, and spiritual. Physical and environmental goals can include recovering from illnesses or ailments, engaging in or mastering a particular physical activity (anything you've ever considered doing), or living or working in a certain place. Mental goals might address career plans, financial objectives, and any limiting beliefs that you'd like to change. Emotional goals have to do with feelings and self-esteem. Social goals are about your relationships with other people, while spiritual objectives have to do with your relationship with God or Spirit. As you do this part of the exercise, ask yourself, "What does my ideal life look like?" "Where do I see myself five or ten years from now?" "What is my purpose—what am I here to do?" Do *not* give yourself a time frame within which to attain any of these goals, and remember, it is *not* necessary to have a plan for getting there.

- **Next, reword all of your goals into affirmations.** For example, a goal might be "I'd like to be free of headaches."

Some simple affirmations might be: *"My headaches are now completely healed"* or *"My headache condition is improving every day."* Then compile a list of about ten affirmations that address your most important goals and desires, and the most limiting beliefs or critical messages that you'd like to change. As you'll read on the following pages, headaches often are triggered by self-criticism. Effective affirmations for headache might also include: *"I love and approve of myself." "I'm always doing the best I can." "I see myself and what I do with eyes of love."*

• **Recite your entire list at least once a day, and whenever you hear a negative, limiting, or critical message, recite the one affirmation that corresponds to that message.** Or you can record them onto a cassette and listen to them in your own voice. Perhaps the most effective method for deriving benefit from affirmations is to *write, recite,* and *visualize* them (see "Guided Imagery and Visualization" below). Using this method, you would write down your affirmation while reciting it aloud, and then close your eyes and imagine what the affirmation looks and/or feels like, engaging as many of your senses as possible. If you can't picture it, it helps to *feel* your affirmations as you recite or write them, since this brings more energy to the experience. Make the process as vivid and real as possible.

I learned this technique from a patient, a man who owns an oil company and works part-time as a psychotherapist. He'd had a terrible case of chronic sinusitis for many years. On our second session, one month into the Sinus Survival Program, I presented this idea of changing some of his limiting, critical, or negative beliefs and clarifying his goals and objectives as a foundation of greater mental health. Shortly after this visit, he formulated a lengthy list of affirmations and goals. Once each day he recited every one of his new beliefs, then wrote them down on a sheet of paper, and after each one he closed his eyes and visualized what that desire or goal would look or feel like. When I next saw him, just over two months later, he told me that he had been repeating this procedure of reciting, writing, and visualizing for sixty consecutive days. He was thrilled to report to me that at least half of his affirmations and goals had already become a reality, including healthy sinuses! He continues to practice this method (using new affirmations) along with the physical and environmental health recommendations that he had implemented at the outset of the program. It is now more than eight years since my third session with him. During that time he has had only two sinus infections, and his chronic sinusitis remains cured.

My patients' affirmation/goal lists provide a blueprint of our work together. The lists also become their personal vision and give direction to their own self-healing process.

You must be able to clarify your desires to have any chance of obtaining them, and as you do this exercise, try to be as specific as possible. The next step is to believe, however minimally, that it is possible for you to meet these goals. The more you repeat the affirmations, the stronger your belief will become.

The third step in this formula for self-realization is *expectation*. (The first step is identifying what you want—*desire;* then, secondly, strengthening the *belief* that it's possible to realize that goal.) The stronger your belief and the more objectives you have already reached, the higher will be your level of expectation. After my chronic sinusitis was cured, I developed the belief that anything is possible, one that has helped me to realize other dreams. Whatever it is that you *desire,* as long as you *believe* it's possible, you can *expect* it to happen. It is not necessary to know how, or to have a definite plan. Just be patient and flexible and be willing to accept the result, even if the "package" in which it arrives is different from what you had envisioned. If your objectives are clear, your intuition will help you make the right decisions to get what you want. Remember that you can always choose what to believe. Rather than continuing with the attitude "I'll believe it when I see it," why not try "When I believe it, then I'll see it."

I've repeatedly seen this technique change lives in a variety of ways other than curing disease. My favorite example is a woman from Tennessee whom I was treating for chronic fatigue, allergies, and sinusitis. In the early years of my holistic practice, I worked with a number of patients long-distance over the phone, never actually meeting them in person. An RN in her fifties, she taught in a nursing school in a small town and had never married, although she wanted to. She had resisted putting marriage on her goal list because, as she explained to me, "I know all the eligible men in town and in my church, and there aren't any possible candidates." I convinced her to include it on her goal list, and her affirmation read simply: *I am happily married.* Within a few months, she received a letter from a former professor of hers with whom she had a friendship years earlier. His wife had died the year before, and he wanted to visit his former student. Within months they were engaged, and a year after beginning her affirmation she was happily married. Her tears of joy over the phone and her gratitude left me in tears as well. We both felt as if we had experienced a miracle.

How you choose to see your headaches or any other chronic condition can play a vital role in the way the disease affects you and whether or not it goes away. Some of the early reactions to a chronic or life-threatening disease are denial ("There must be some mistake"), anger and frustration ("Why me?" "What terrible luck"), self-pity ("I'll never be able to enjoy life again"), and resignation ("I'll just have to put up with it and continue to live this way for the rest of my life"). All of these are quite normal and understandable responses to something as devastating as an incurable condition. However, if you are interested in healing yourself, it is important to get beyond this point and look at your disease in a different light. According to Bernie Siegel, who contributed the following material to the book *Chop Wood, Carry Water,* you have several choices:

- **Accept your illness.** Being resigned to an illness can be destructive and can allow the illness to run your life, but accepting it allows energy to be freed for other things in your life.
- **See the illness as a source of growth.** If you begin to grow psychologically in response to the loss the illness has

created in your life, then you don't need to have a physical illness anymore.

- **View your illness as a positive redirection in your life.** This means that you don't have to judge anything that happens to you. If you get fired from a job, for example, assume that you are being redirected toward something else you are supposed to be doing. Your entire life changes when you say that something is just a redirection. You are then at peace. Everything is okay and you go on your way, knowing that the new direction is the one that is intrinsically right for you. After a while, you begin to *feel* that this is true.

- **Death or recurrence of illness is no longer seen as synonymous with failure after the aforementioned steps are accomplished, but simply as further choices or steps.** If staying alive were your sole goal, you would have to be a failure because you do have to die someday. However, when you begin to accept the inevitability of death and see that you have only a limited time, you begin to realize that you might as well enjoy the present to the best of your ability.

- **Learn self-love and peace of mind, and the body responds.** Your body gets "live" or "energy" messages when you say "I love myself." That's not the ego talking, it's self-esteem. It's as if someone else is loving you, saying that you are a worthwhile person, believing in you, and telling you that you are here to give something to the world. When you do that, your immune system says, "This person likes living; let's fight for his or her life."

- **Don't make physical change your sole goal.** Seek peace of mind, acceptance, and forgiveness. Learn to love. In the process, the disease won't be totally overlooked: It will be seen as one of the problems you are having, and perhaps one of your fears. If you learn about hope, love, acceptance, forgiveness, and peace of mind, the disease may go away in the process.

- **Achieve immortality through love.** The only way you can live forever is to love somebody. Then you can really leave a gift behind. When you live that way, as many people with physical illnesses do, it is even possible to decide when you die. You can say, "Thank you, I've used my body to its limit. I have loved as much as I possibly can, and I'm leaving at two o'clock today." And you go. Then maybe you have spent half an hour dying and the rest of your life living; but when these things are not done, you may spend a lot of your life dying, and only a little living.

I realize that you will not die from your headaches, but each of these options for looking at physical illness can work for you as a form of preventive medicine. In my experience, incapacitating pain and imminent death have provided the greatest motivation for people to change, but why wait until you have reached that point of crisis?

EMOTIONAL CAUSES OF HEADACHE

Although there is no specific **migraine** personality, from his many years of experience in working with several thousand patients with migraine, Dr. Ken Peters has found the majority of migraineurs to be *perfectionists* while setting very high goals for themselves. Along with perfectionism comes the fear of making mistakes. They often take care of others to the extent of *self-sacrifice,* in which they become both physically and emotionally depleted. They have a difficult time *saying no* to requests for their services from others, tend to take on a great deal of responsibility, and find it difficult to delegate to others ("no one will do the job as well as I can"). Often they keep long lists of tasks they need to accomplish each day and feel guilty if they don't accomplish them all. They seem to have a *lack of joy* in their lives. Migraineurs are not the prototypical type A personalities since they are not competitive with others, but they often tend to push themselves beyond their healthy limits. They tend to chronically overdo, worry about the lists that are piling up and not getting done, and go into *deep feelings of being overwhelmed.* This creates a vicious cycle of physical and emotional stress and fatigue, which

will often trigger a disabling headache. It's almost as if the headache serves the purpose of forcing the migraineur to slow down
and temporarily pull away from the pressures and responsibilities
of everyday life. The symptoms of sensitivity to light, sound,
smell, and movement forces the migraineur to pull back into a
state of isolation. In fact, the severity of symptoms forces the
sufferer to take time off and be still. When one is in excessive
doing mode the sympathetic nervous system, or doing branch of
the nervous system, is cranking at a high rate. The migraine can
come on when there is an abrupt shift from sympathetic nervous
system dominance to parasympathetic dominance; parasympathetic is the relaxation branch of the nervous system. It's like
cruising at high speed, pedal-to-the-metal, and abruptly hitting
the breaks with both feet. This is the critical time when blood
vessels violently dilate. In the attempt to balance from doing to
relaxation mode, the nervous system overcompensates. This is
why most migraines start in the early-morning hours of sleep.
Most sufferers wake up, or are awakened by, a migraine. Sleep
and rest is vital to recovery once you are able to sleep. I recommend scheduling time to be still before you are forced to do so!
Regular periods of meditation and complete physical stillness—
hopefully on a daily basis—can train your nervous system to
smoothly transition from sympathetic to parasympathetic mode,
the result being a better pacing of nervous energy.

While the symptom of headache is being suppressed with
medication, it can provide you the opportunity to heighten
your awareness of the possible emotional factors that triggered
it, and to help you to see where your life is imbalanced. Many
migraineurs have come to the realization that they are lacking in
self-nurturing. One helpful technique for strengthening this aspect of your life is to make a list of ten things that you enjoy
doing (refer to page 171). These should be simple activities, such
as going to a movie or reading a magazine. Then do one of these
things each day. If you're a migraineur who already creates daily
"to do" lists, then put one of these enjoyable activities high on

that list, so you are sure to get to it. If you feel guilty doing these pleasurable tasks, just consider them part of your doctor's prescription! You must also realize it is OK to say no to others' requests for your time and energy. Practice doing this, and acknowledge yourself whenever you've succeeded. Keep in mind that if you push yourself too far or take on too much, it will very often trigger a migraine that will prevent you from maintaining all of your responsibilities, both at home and at work.

By learning to pace yourself, you'll establish healthier limits with respect to taking on new projects and responsibilities, and you'll be practicing self-nurturing. This healing process involves getting adequate rest and sleep, delegating responsibilities to others both at home and at work, and being satisfied with what you have accomplished each day instead of feeling guilty about not completing all the tasks on your daily list of things to do. You can work hard, but it must be balanced with play and relaxation. Ask yourself what your headache is symbolically telling you about your lifestyle, so that it can help direct you toward a life of greater balance. This process of increased self-awareness and re-balancing is essential to significantly reduce the frequency and intensity of your headaches and to experience optimal health!

I have recently begun formal training to become certified as a Healing Touch (HT) practitioner. HT is an energy-based therapeutic approach to healing that uses touch to influence the bioenergy system that exists in and around the human body. This technique can have a profound effect upon physical, emotional, mental, and spiritual health. It is based in large part on the energy centers, or chakras ("spinning wheel" in Sanskrit), as they are known in Ayurvedic medicine. The foundation of that healing system is the understanding that we are spiritual/energy beings, and that there are seven major chakras that form an energy matrix that supports physical-mental-emotional-spiritual life. Each of these seven chakras reflects various aspects of consciousness, is associated with different mental and emotional issues, and corresponds to specific body parts and organs. Every physical dysfunction or disease relates primarily to one or two of the chakras.

While working and training with Janna Moll, a gifted practitioner and teacher of healing touch and energetic healing, I have observed her, on several occasions, rapidly and completely relieve the pain of a migraine attack. Among other things, she has helped me to appreciate the extent of the connection between mind and body through the chakra system, and the specificity of the emotional factors contributing to physical problems. For example, *tension* headaches are energetically related to the throat chakra that is located at the suprasternal notch at the base of the throat. Compromise or weakening of a chakra results from anything that prevents the energy from flowing at its optimum. Compromise of the throat chakra can lead to a tightening of all muscles in the upper back, shoulders, jaw, and neck, resulting in tension headaches.

The underlying mental/emotional issues of the throat chakra are about communication, and how we communicate with the world. Therefore, the issues around speaking your truth (speaking from your heart), sharing your ideas, and expressing your creativity should be investigated. Have you said what you need to say? Are you holding yourself back from expressing your truth? Additionally, there is a close association between the throat chakra and the sacral chakra, or our emotional center located in the lower abdomen about two inches below the belly button. This adds the component of feelings as a contributing factor to tension headaches. Have you shared how you feel? Are you holding back your tears or joy? By investigating the underlying emotional situation that is not being expressed, we can clear the *tension* being created in the energetic system. The longer compromise exists in these energy centers, the more likely tension headaches will become chronic.

Migraine headaches are governed primarily by the brow chakra or intuitive energy center located in the lower forehead. The factors contributing to migraine are important indicators of what the mental and emotional issues are that underlie the condition. In most cases of migraine, the intuitive aspects of the migraineur are compromised. However, I do know some people who have chosen to use their experience of the migraine to deepen their intuitive insight. For example, Dr. Todd Nelson often writes poetry as he emerges from an episode of migraine. Additionally, there is a close association between migraines and the crown chakra, located in the top of the head. This energy center governs our relationship with the Divine (God or Spirit).

The following are some examples of the chakra issues related to several of the migraine triggers:

Food allergies—I should not be here (this life, this planet, this family, etc.). It is not okay to nourish myself. I must punish myself, or be punished for living. I cannot have joy in life.

Stress—Life is not pleasant. Life is painful and/or hopeless. I am here against my will. God has abandoned me.

Hormonal—It is not okay to be intuitive. My intuitions are dangerous or forbidden. I cannot see or hear the truth. I must suffer because I am a woman/man.

Constriction or compromise in the brow chakra will impact the higher issues of communication (throat chakra), such as "I cannot think clearly" or "I lack understanding (intuition) about what is going on." Compromise of the brow and crown chakras is most closely aligned with understanding our association with the Divine, our place in the world, and life's meaning on a spiritual level. Why do good people suffer? Why is life so hard? Why did God abandon me/us/them? (God is not just.) Sleep and deeper spiritual wisdom, purpose and optimism, will be disrupted with compromise of the brow and crown chakras. The longer compromise exists in these energy centers, the longer the duration of the migraine and the more frequently it will occur.

Cluster headaches are governed by the solar plexus, brow, and crown chakras. The belief in energetic healing is that these headaches are often a result of a head injury or head trauma (sometimes occurring many years before). Their severity results in a dramatic compromise to the energy centers. Often there are leaks in the energy field encompassing the head, causing a variety of symptoms that can fluctuate over time. Unlike a migraine, the most effective treatment is to determine the location of these energy leaks and seal them in order to facilitate healing. But similar to migraine, if the symptoms are untreated they can worsen over time and create a cellular memory of pain, resulting in severe "multiple migraines."

Interestingly, men are the predominant sufferers of cluster headaches. The major reason energetically is the involvement of the solar plexus chakra. This chakra is located in the abdomen about two inches above the belly button and is energetically where issues of abuse, addictions, control, egotism, and poor self-esteem are located. Our personal power resides here. The related issues of solar plexus involvement in cluster headaches might include: I am no longer in control of my life. I am not doing, or going where I want to. I am no longer important (in my job, family, community, etc.). I have to suffer to be in control. I have to control my anger. Life is too serious to enjoy. I deserve to suffer because . . .

Energetically, all three types of headaches can have an inherited component. Many times it is not directly obvious how, but is related to the compromised chakras and their issues. The greater and longer the compromise to the energetic system, the greater the intensity and chronicity of the headaches and general dis-ease. Ms. Moll believes that by clearing the energy system, investigating the underlying issues, and working with your health care provider, most incidences of headache can be greatly diminished or eliminated.

Louise Hay, in *You Can Heal Your Life,* states that the probable emotional cause of headaches has to do with: invalidating the self; self-criticism; and fear.

GUIDED IMAGERY AND VISUALIZATION

Visualization is a skill all of us have and one that we use every day. Most of the time, however, we do so unconsciously, such as when we daydream. The fifty thousand thoughts we have each and every day are often accompanied by inner pictures, or imagery, with corresponding emotions. Since the 1970s, researchers, physicians, and other health care professionals have been examining how to harness these mental images in order to use them consciously to create improved states of well-being. Due to their continued work, thousands of individuals nationwide are learning how to use visualization and guided imagery to enhance their health. In many cases their results have been astounding. Since 1971, radiation oncologist O. Carl Simonton, M.D. has been a pioneer in developing imagery as a self-care tool for cancer patients to use to bolster their response rate to traditional cancer treatments, with remarkable success. The first patient to whom he taught his techniques was a sixty-one-year-old man who had been diagnosed with a "hopeless" case of throat cancer. In conjunction with his radiation treatments, the man spent five to fifteen minutes three times a day imagining himself healthy. Within two months he was completely cancer-free.

A similarly remarkable case is that of Garrett Porter, a patient of Patricia Norris, Ph.D., another leader in the field of guided imagery. Garrett was nine and had been diagnosed with an inoperable brain tumor. Using biofeedback techniques in conjunction with imagery based on Garrett's favorite TV show, *Star Trek* (he pictured missiles striking and destroying his tumor), Garrett was able to completely reverse his condition within a year, with brain scans confirming his tumor's disappearance. He subsequently wrote a book about his healing entitled *Why Me?*

Numerous studies also confirm the health benefits of imagery and visualization. For example, college volunteers who practiced imagery twice daily for six weeks experienced a marked increase in salivary immunoglobulin A as compared to a control group who did not practice imagery. In another study, the well-known drop in helper T-immune cells in students facing the stress of final examinations was greatly reduced in a group utilizing relaxation and imagery each day for a month before exams. And patients scheduled for gallbladder surgery who listened to imagery tapes before and after their operations had less wound inflammation, lower cortisone levels, and less anxiety than did controls who were treated with comparable periods of quiet only.

Like most of the other therapies outlined in this chapter, one of the most exciting things about guided imagery and visualization is that both techniques are powerful self-healing tools that can be used to create positive change in almost any area of your life. Besides physical health, imagery can help you feel more peaceful and relaxed, assist you in further developing your creative talents, create more fulfillment in your relationships, improve your ability to achieve career goals, and dissolve negative habit patterns. All that is necessary is a commitment to practice the techniques on a regular basis.

Guided imagery and visualization work to improve and maintain health because of their ability to directly affect our bodies at a cellular level, particularly with regard to neuropeptides. In addition, the use of imagery can often provide greater insight into causes and treatment for chronic conditions, guiding us toward the most personalized and effective solutions for our particular health problems. This occurs because our mental images are so deeply connected to our emotions, which, as we have discussed, are usually interconnected with the events in our lives. By using imagery, you can become better aware of what emotional issues may lie beneath the surface of your life and begin the process of healing them.

There are two types of guided imagery and visualization: preconceived or preselected images employed by you or your health care professional in order to address a specific problem and achieve a specific outcome, such as healing migraine, and imagery that occurs spontaneously as you sit comfortably, eyes closed and breathing freely. Both forms have value, so try them both and see which works best for you. What follows are two techniques you can use to make imagery a part of your Headache Survival Program. The first is a form of guided imagery, while the latter is conducive for allowing spontaneous imagery to occur on its own.

The Remembrance Technique. This exercise can be adapted to improve issues or conditions in any area of your life. It's called the Remembrance Technique because in our core selves we are already whole. In many respects, healing is simply a remembrance of that state in order to reconnect with it. Begin this exercise by sitting comfortably in a chair or lying down in bed. Select a time and place when you will not be disturbed. Close your eyes and focus on your breathing. Take a few deep, unforced breaths to help you relax. With each inhalation, imagine that soothing, relaxing energy is flowing through all areas of your body. As you exhale, visualize the cares and concerns of the day gradually disappearing. Do this for two or three minutes, allowing your breath to carry you to a place of calm relaxation.

Now choose the issue you want to focus on for the rest of the exercise, and recall a time when the outcome you desire was something you have already experienced. For example, if you have migraine, remember a time when you were in excellent health and never had the slightest worry (even in the deepest recesses of your mind) about the sudden onset of an incapacitating headache. Allow yourself to reexperience that time, using all of your senses to make what you are imagining as vivid as possible. Once you have reconnected to the experience, bring it into the present *as if it were actually happening now*. Stay with the experience for at least five more minutes, mentally affirming that you *are* experiencing the state you desire here in the present.

Another form of preselected imagery is to focus on an image of healthy blood vessels surrounding your brain, with the perfect level of patency (opening)—neither too dilated nor constricted, relaxed muscles lining the blood vessels, and the optimum amount of both oxygen and serotonin flowing through the bloodstream (these could be represented by a radiant white light. As you picture this, you are taking deep belly breaths and feeling all of your tight muscles relax. (This particular imagery can be practiced for either migraine or tension headache. With the latter type I would suggest primarily picturing scalp, neck, and shoulder muscles relaxing, even at the tissue level.) Prepare yourself in the same way I've described above—sitting, relaxed, and focused on breath. Even though this is a preselected image (like Garrett Porter's missiles striking his tumor), it can also be a dynamic process in which the image changes and evolves with each session of imagery. You might see a radiant white light filling every cell in the muscle tissue of your neck, shoulders, and upper back. Or another time you might picture a guardian angel or spirit guide gently and compassionately caressing your head, face, and neck. Allow your imagery to be creative without placing any restrictions upon it. There is no one correct image to use for healing headaches. Whatever works for you and feels good is the "right" image.

Spontaneous Imagery. In this exercise, instead of preselecting a specific outcome, you are going to allow your own unconscious to communicate with you through imagery about whatever situation in your life you choose to focus on. As in the preceding exercise, sit or lie down comfortably in a quiet place, close your eyes, and focus on your breath until you feel yourself settling into a deeper state of relaxation. Now focus on the physical problem you'd like to heal or the area in your life into which you desire to gain greater insight, allowing thoughts and images to freely and spontaneously emerge. Although you may have chosen your headaches to focus on, you may be surprised by what you experience, but don't judge it. Trust that your unconscious knows what you most need to understand, and allow your imagery to lead you to that answer. Continue this exercise for five to ten minutes, and when you complete it, write down what you experienced so that you can contemplate it for possible further insight. As a variation to this exercise, you can first ask a question of yourself, such as "Why do I have headaches?" or "What do I have to learn from my migraine?" and then see what image appears. From there, you may find yourself engaged in a dialog between yourself and your unconscious that results in answers and solutions you did not know were possible.

When you first begin to practice mental imagery techniques, don't be discouraged if at first "nothing seems to be happening." Like any new skill, achieving results in imagery takes time. Remember that the language of your unconscious, like the symbolism of your dreams, is usually not literal or rational. It may take some time before you are able to grasp the messages of the images you perceive. Keeping a written log of your experience can make learning this new "language" easier.

BIOFEEDBACK AND RELAXATION

Studies have shown that learning and regularly practicing biofeedback or any of the relaxation approaches achieves a 45 to 80 percent reduction or elimination in both migraine headache severity and frequency. Most headache clinics offer this service, providing a biofeedback therapist who acts as a coach to help you to master this potentially highly therapeutic technique.

The essence of *biofeedback* is to learn how to encounter stress without adverse physiologic effects—that is, muscle tension, rapid heart rate and respiration, perspiration, or lowered body temperature. A typical course of biofeedback consists of eight to ten weekly 30- to 45-minute sessions. Learning to control body functions such as temperature occurs through *muscle relaxation,* which is achieved through progressive relaxation, visualization, and breathing techniques. Both techniques—biofeedback and muscle relaxation—can be taught by a skilled practitioner and are not difficult to learn. However, the key to your success in preventing and treating your headaches lies in the daily practice of these techniques. The practice sessions can be a few seconds or minutes long, but they have to be very frequent. A conscious effort is required in the first few weeks of training, but gradually these very brief relaxation techniques can become a subconscious habit. It can be quite helpful in relieving tension throughout the day, which in turn will reduce the frequency of headaches.

Children are especially quick learners of biofeedback and can often learn to prevent their migraines in only four to five sessions. In some cases they are able to stop their headache once it begins.

Hypnosis is also a successful therapeutic modality for treating migraine. Self-hypnosis can be particularly helpful in children and teenagers.

OPTIMISM AND HUMOR

In the Bible it is written: "A cheerful heart is good medicine, but a downcast spirit dries up the bones" (Proverbs 17:22). Science is now beginning to verify this ancient truth, revealing that optimism and humor are integral factors in one's overall health, providing both physical and mental benefits. One of the most famous anecdotes illustrating this point concerns Norman Cousins, who in his book *Anatomy of an Illness* attributed his recovery from ankylosing spondylitis (a potentially crippling arthritic condition of the spine) to the many hours he spent watching Marx Brothers movies and reruns of *Candid Camera* while taking megadoses of vitamin C. The more he laughed, the more his pain diminished, until eventually his illness completely disappeared, never to return. Based on his experience with humor, Cousins went on to explore mind-body medicine at UCLA. Today a number of institutions are studying the healing potential of humor, such as the appropriately named Gesundheit Institute in Arlington, Virginia, founded and directed by Patch Adams, M.D.

Some of the most in-depth research in this area has been conducted by Robert Ornstein, Ph.D., and David Sobel, M.D., who presented their findings in their book *Healthy Pleasures.* They discovered that the people who are optimally healthy also tend to be optimistic and happy, and possess the belief that things will work out no matter what their difficulties may be. Such people maintain a vital sense of humor about life and enjoy a good laugh, often at their own expense. According to Ornstein and Sobel, they also expect good things of life, including being liked and respected by others, and experience pleasure in most of what they do. They usually look at stressful situations as temporary setbacks, specific to the immediate circumstance and due largely to external causes. Pessimists, on the other hand, when faced with life-challenging events, tend to think they will be permanent ("It's going to last forever"), generalize the problem to their whole lives ("It's going to spoil everything"), and blame themselves ("It's my fault"). Recent research at the Mayo Clinic suggests that pessimism is a significant risk factor for early death. More than 800 patients were given a personality test that categorized them as optimistic, mixed, or pessimistic. After their health status was evaluated thirty years later, the pessimists had a significantly higher-than-expected death rate.

Optimistic people also tend to laugh a lot, something that most likely plays an important role in their health. Studies have shown that laughter can strengthen the immune system. One study, for instance, found that test subjects who watched videotapes of the comedian Richard Pryor produced increased levels of antibodies in their saliva. Furthermore, subjects in the study who said they frequently used humor to cope with life stress had consistently higher baseline levels of those antibodies that help to combat infections such as colds.

Hearty laughter is actually a form of gentle exercise, or "inner jogging." Describing the physiological effects of laughter, Ornstein and Sobel write:

A robust laugh gives the muscles of your face, shoulders, diaphragm, and abdomen a good workout. With convulsive or side-splitting laughter, even your arm and leg muscles come into play. Your heart rate and blood pressure temporarily rise, breathing becomes faster and deeper, and oxygen surges through your bloodstream. A vigorous laugh can burn up as many calories per hour as brisk walking or cycling.

The afterglow of a hearty laugh is positively relaxing. Blood pressure may temporarily fall, your muscles go limp, and you bask in a mild euphoria. Some researchers speculate that laughter triggers the release of endorphins, the brain's own opiates; this may account for the pain relief and euphoria that accompany laughter.

In short, laughter's benefits are many and profound. Unfortunately most of us don't laugh enough. One study found that young children laugh about 400 times a day, while the average adult only 14 times. When the question posed to octogenarians is "If you had your life to live over again, what would you do differently?" the answer often is "I'd take life much less seriously." Comedian George Burns, who lived to the age of one hundred, wrote the book *Wisdom of the 90's* at age ninety-five. He attributed his ability to laugh at himself as well as loving what he did for a living as the most important factors in his longevity.

Both optimism and a sense of humor are directly related to our beliefs. If you wish to become more optimistic and experience more humor and fun in your life, practice the exercises outlined in this chapter. It may take time before you achieve the results you desire, but your commitment will prove well worth it and will impact your mood, mental health, and even survival. Nothing quite epitomizes the free flow of life-force energy as much as laughter, and all of us can stand to laugh even more than we do. Be advised, however. There is one side effect to this powerful form of self-healing: more pleasure.

EMOTIONAL HEALTH

The emotionally fit are able to identify their feelings and can express, fully experience, and accept them as well. I have heard contemporary American culture referred to as the "no-feeling" society. The feelings are certainly present, but as a result of our lifestyle we have constructed such formidable protective barriers around ourselves that to a great extent we have become unconscious of our feelings, especially the more uncomfortable ones.

There are those who believe there are only two basic human emotions: love and fear. The so-called negative or painful emotions, such as anger, grief, anxiety, depression, envy, guilt, hatred, hostility, jealousy, loneliness, shame, and worry, are all expressions of fear. The feelings of acceptance, intimacy, joy, power, approval, and peacefulness are all aspects of love. The greater our degree of fear, the less capable we are of experiencing love.

With any chronic condition or illness, including headaches, fear becomes the predominant emotion. When this occurs, your greatest liability is your *loss of love*—for yourself and those closest to you. It becomes a much greater challenge to nurture yourself and to feel fully alive when you're consumed with the anxiety and insecurity created by your ongoing physical discomfort and disability.

Some mental health professionals consider four basic emotions: love or joy, sadness, anger, and fear. So at any given moment you're feeling either glad, sad, mad, or scared, or some combination of these. In our culture it is not socially acceptable to express most of the "negative" emotions, and men especially are not supposed to show signs of weakness or insecurity or to cry ("Big boys don't cry"). The majority of us have learned to repress these feelings until we are unaware that we even have them. Society has helped us suppress our painful (negative) feelings by perpetuating the myth of an emotionally pain-free existence. The numerous ads in the media for analgesics to treat the pain of headaches and arthritis, and the common use of alcohol or drugs to dull the pain of an awkward social situation or personal crisis give us the clear message that *not only is pain a bad thing, but life can be pain free.*

If we spend less time avoiding emotional pain, but instead focus our attention on it, accept it, and relax into it, the pain would diminish or even disappear. *If we continue to ignore and repress it, it often manifests itself as physical pain, illness, or disease.* Redford Williams, M.D., a researcher in behavioral medicine at the Duke University Medical Center, has gathered a wealth of data suggesting that chronic anger is so damaging to the body that it ranks with, or even exceeds, cigarette smoking, obesity, and a high-fat diet as a powerful risk factor for early death. Williams reported that people who scored high on a hostility scale as teenagers were much more likely than their more cheer-ful peers to have elevated cholesterol levels as adults, suggesting a link between unremitting anger and heart disease.

In another study, Dr. Mara Julius, an epidemiologist at the University of Michigan, analyzed the effects of chronic anger on women over a period of eighteen years. She found that women who had answered initial test questions with obvious signs of long-term, suppressed anger were three times more likely to have *died* during the study than those women who did not harbor such hostile feelings. Chronic sinusitis is usually asso-ciated with a tremendous amount of unexpressed anger, and I've also found it to be the primary trigger for most colds and sinus infections, as well as being an important contributing fac-tor to headache, arthritis, and many other chronic conditions.

Clyde Reid is director of the Center for New Beginnings in Denver. In his insightful book *Celebrate the Temporary*, he says, "Leaning into life's pain can also be a lifestyle, and is far more satisfying than the avoidance style. It requires small doses of plain courage to look pain in the eye, but it prepares you for more serious pain when it comes. In the meantime, all the en-ergy expended to avoid pain is now available for the business of living."

I am not advocating that you seek out painful experiences, nor am I proposing that you endure prolonged or persistent pain. That is called suffering. Health and happiness do not have prerequisites that require you to suffer. Life is to be enjoyed, but the notion that it can be lived entirely without painful feelings is an unhealthy belief. Pain and joy are intertwined, and ***the more you allow yourself to accept, embrace, and feel both pain and joy, the greater will be your sense of emotional health.***

Of the mental-emotional connection, Albert Ellis, a psychol-ogist and founder of the Institute for Rational-Emotive Ther-apy in New York City, has said that "virtually all 'emotionally disturbed' individuals actually think crookedly, magically, dog-matically, and unrealistically." David D. Bums, M.D., a psychia-trist and author of *The Feeling Good Handbook,* writes:

Certain kinds of negative thoughts make people unhappy. In fact, I believe that unhealthy, negative emotions—depression, anxiety, excessive anger, inappropriate guilt, etc.—are *always* caused by illogical, distorted thoughts, even if those thoughts may seem absolutely valid at the time. By learning to look at things more realistically, by getting rid of your distorted thinking patterns, you can break out of a bad mood, often in a short period of time, without having to rely on medication or prolonged psychotherapy.

Burns offers the following list of thought distortions:

- **All-or-nothing thinking.** You classify things into absolute, black-and-white categories.
- **Overgeneralization.** You view a single negative situation as a never-ending pattern of defeat.
- **Mental filtering.** You dwell on negatives and overlook positives.
- **Discounting the positive.** You insist your accomplishments or positive qualities "don't count."
- **Magnification or minimization.** You blow things out of proportion or shrink their importance inappropriately.
- **Making *should* statements.** You criticize yourself and others by using the terms *should, shouldn't, must, ought,* and *have to.*
- **Emotional reasoning.** You reason from how you feel. If you feel like an idiot, you assume you must be one. If you don't feel like doing something, you put it off.
- **Jumping to conclusions.** You "mind-read," assuming, without definite evidence of it, that people are reacting negatively to you. Or you "fortune-tell," arbitrarily predicting bad outcomes.
- **Labeling.** You identify with your shortcomings. Instead of saying, "I made a mistake," you tell yourself, "I'm such a jerk . . . a real loser."
- **Personalization and blame.** You blame yourself for something you weren't entirely responsible for, or you blame others and ignore the impact of your own attitudes or behavior.

As I've already said, negative thoughts and the feelings they engender contribute to physical illness. The perfectionism, self-sacrificing, lack of joy and self-nurturing, and fear of making mistakes experienced by many people with migraine are frequently associated with several of the thought distortions listed above. These repeated thoughts will often trigger anger (ultimately with ourselves) and depression (almost always fueled by repressed anger), which, if not expressed, can cause further imbalance in serotonin metabolism and aggravate migraine. Many of these same critical and limiting messages are also preventing you from achieving your goals and seeing your "wish list" become a reality. These theories of Drs. Ellis and Burns constitute the foundation of *cognitive psychotherapy*—the form of counseling I've found to be highly effective for many patients with both migraine and tension headache.

One self-care approach you might try for gaining greater self-awareness is to attempt to identify the mental and emotional issues that may have contributed to causing your headache. Other than the concepts described on page 178 related to the chakra system and energy healing, one method I've used with my patients for many years is to consider the possible benefits or secondary gain resulting from having this condition. They may not be readily apparent, but if you're open to this introspective exploration you'll usually find some answers, however minimal, to the question "What are the benefits of having this migraine?" As I've previously mentioned, one possible result of having this incapacitating headache is that you get to rest or sleep in a dark, quiet room with no stimulation. Perhaps this is the extent of self-nurturing that you've needed but weren't able to provide yourself unless you were disabled by the headache. Other possible gains may include "My husband [or wife] pays more attention to me"; "I don't have to work or exercise"; "I'm no longer expected to perform at the level I had been [perfection], and that has reduced a lot of pressure [stress] that I'd been feeling." Whether it's more attention, a need for nurturing, job dissatisfaction, performance anxiety, or some other unmet need, I believe there are almost always some secondary gains associated with every chronic condition. Since you did not respond preventively, in order to meet those unconscious needs, your body created an illness or an incapacitating pain. If these not-so-subtle benefits can be understood and you become more aware of what your needs and desires are, it will help considerably in identifying the emotional causes of your physical problem and allow you to work on resolving them. Once you have become aware of the issues, you can then begin expressing your emotions while addressing the unmet needs your feelings have revealed. The process continues with acceptance: knowing that it's okay to feel whatever you're feeling. This healing process will not only lead you to emotional health, it will help you practice preventive medicine, and will also take you a giant step closer to being free of your headaches. Remember, a basic tenet of mind-body medicine is that *your core issues are held in your tissues.*

BREATHWORK AND MEDITATION

The benefits of learning to breathe properly and consciously (see breathing exercises on page 81) go far beyond the physical. Proper breathing can also improve your mood, make you mentally more alert, and help you to become more aware of deeply held and often painful feelings. Most important, by working with your breathing, you can begin to heal the wounded, rejected, unnurtured, unloved, unacknowledged, and disowned parts of yourself and bring them into wholeness.

The primary reason so many of us breathe unconsciously and inefficiently lies in the fact that our breathing process began traumatically at birth. We were forcibly expelled from the security of the womb and compelled to take our first breath on our own when we encountered the outside world. Often that first breath came as a harsh and unexpected shock, accompanied by pain and confusion. In order to suppress such pain, newborns typically follow their first inhalation by pausing and holding their breath for a moment as they struggle to make sense of their new environment. Today a number of researchers in the field of mental health speculate that this first pause in our breath not only sets the stage for a lifetime of shallow, inefficient breathing but also conditions us to suppress our painful emotions instead of learning how to accept and relax into them. You can observe this pattern in yourself the next time you find yourself feeling shock, fear, pain, or worry. If you take a moment to observe yourself in the initial experience of such emotions, more than likely you will find that you are also holding your breath or breathing very shallowly, or perhaps even wheezing.

Breathwork, also known as "breath therapy," is a means of learning how to breathe consciously and fully in order to deal with emotional pain more effectively and healthfully. There are many approaches to breathwork, ranging from ancient breathing techniques found in the traditions of *yoga, tai chi,* and *qigong,* to modern-day methods such as *rebirthing* (also known as *conscious connected breathing),* developed by Leonard Orr, and *holotropic breathwork,* developed by Stanislav Grof. All of them have in common a focus on the breath and the ability to move energy through the body and connect you with suppressed emotions and limiting beliefs in order to heal them.

Most breathwork therapies use the technique of connected breathing, first pioneered by Leonard Orr. In connected breathing, each inhalation immediately follows the exhalation of the preceding breath without pause. (Typically we breathe unconsciously, pausing between inhalation and exhalation.) The pattern of respiration can vary according to technique. Sometimes it is rapid; sometimes it is deep, slow, and full. In addition, some approaches recommend breathing in and out through the mouth, instead of the nose, and both abdominal and chest breathing can be used. In rebirthing, sometimes the therapy is performed in a tub or underwater with the use of a snorkel, although this usually does not occur until after the client has had a number of "dry" connected breathing sessions and has become comfortable with the movement of energy and integration of emotions that commonly occur during the rebirthing process. Because of the emotional release that can result from breathwork, it is advisable to learn the techniques under the direction of a skilled breath therapist. Once you gain proficiency, however, you will have at your disposal a powerful self-healing technique that you can practice daily on your own.

Meditation also offers a multitude of emotional health benefits, as well as significant headache improvment—both migraine and tension. The regular practice of meditation can potentially eliminate or reduce the need for medication. There are numerous meditation techniques, but all of them can be accurately described as conscious breathing methods. Meditation's many documented physiological benefits include improved relief from chronic pain and headache; immune function; reduced stress, including decreased levels of adrenaline, cortisone, and free radicals; increased oxygen intake; lower blood pressure and heart rate; and a reduction of core body temperature, which has been linked to increased longevity. Among the psychological benefits of meditation are greater relaxation; improved focus on the present instead of regrets and worries about the past and future; enhanced creativity and cognitive functioning, heightened spiritual awareness (including insights leading to the healing of past emotional trauma); improved awareness and management of beliefs and emotions; and a greater compassion and recognition of others and oneself as parts of a greater whole.

The following is a simple meditation technique that utilizes breathing to promote mental calm. Select a quiet place and sit in a chair with your back straight and your feet on the floor. Close your eyes and begin abdominal or belly breathing, inhaling and exhaling through your nose at a rate of three to four full breaths (inhale and exhale) per minute. The object of this exercise is to stay focused on your breath, allowing whatever thoughts you have to come and go without being absorbed by them. Should you find your attention wandering, bring it back to your breath. You can also enhance the process by silently repeating a short affirmation, or a positive phrase, such as *God, love,* or *peace,* on both the inhale and the exhale. At first, try to do this exercise for five minutes once or twice a day, gradually working up to twenty minutes twice daily. Don't be discouraged if at first you find this exercise difficult to practice. For most Americans, sitting and breathing without thinking or external stimulation is not easy. With time and continued practice, especially in the morning and before you go to bed, you will begin to notice the benefits meditation affords. (For more on meditation, see Chapter 6.)

DEALING WITH ANGER

Unexpressed anger, or anger that is expressed inappropriately, is both harmful and extremely common in our society. Most of us were taught very early in life that anger was an unacceptable emotion. When it was expressed, it often elicited fear in us, and was usually equated with bodily harm and loss of control ("He's really lost it"; "He's out of control"). This inability to safely express anger has been shown to produce many serious health consequences, from heart attacks to headaches. Today many psychotherapists are combining sound and body movement techniques to help their patients deal with their anger, finding that such approaches can be far more effective than simply talking about it. The following techniques can be safely employed by anyone to release the highly charged emotional energy of anger. They are most effective when employed regularly as preventive measures, instead of allowing anger to build up into a state of chronic, health-impacting tension, much less explosive rage.

Screaming
This is the most common anger-release technique due to the fact that all of us already know how to do it. In his novel *Tai-Pan,* author James Clavell wrote that the chieftains of ancient Scotland for centuries maintained the custom of "the screaming tree." From the time they entered adolescence, males of the clan were instructed to go into the forest and select a tree to which they could express their discontent. Then, whenever their troubles grew too great to otherwise deal with, they would go to the

forest alone and scream with the tree as their witness until their emotions settled.

The value of screaming is no secret to young children, who commonly scream when they are greatly upset, only to exhibit a smiling face moments afterward. For adults, the biggest difficulty involved is finding a place to scream in privacy. Screaming when you are home alone, in the basement or closet, in the car with the windows up, or in a secluded spot outside are all possibilities. To get the most benefit, take a deep abdominal breath before you scream, and then direct the scream from your diaphragm or deep within your chest cavity, as this will protect your vocal cords. As you scream, slowly move your upper body from side to side or up and down. Usually, after two or three screams in succession, you will begin to feel much better.

The angry letter (not sent)

This technique is increasingly employed by therapists to help their clients release their anger. It involves writing a letter to the person with whom you are angry, listing all of the reasons why you are upset with them. As you write, allow yourself to express whatever comes to mind, no matter how harsh or offensive it may seem. Once the letter is written, read it over, and if anything else occurs to you that you wish to express, write that down, too, before signing it. Then either burn the letter or tear it up into small pieces.

Punching

Punching a bag, pillow, or sofa is another effective method of dissipating anger. Remember to grunt or yell with each punch. A variation of this method is to take hold of a pillow and hit it against the floor, sofa, or wall. With either approach, it takes only a few moments before you will start to feel your anger transforming into satisfaction and even joy. Remember, anger, in and of itself, is not a negative emotion to be shunned. It's only when it remains bottled up inside of us unexpressed that it becomes unhealthy. *Safely and appropriately expressing your anger in socially acceptable ways can dramatically improve the way you feel, both emotionally and physically.*

However, simply venting anger doesn't do the whole job. In fact, one study in April 1999 concluded that punching to release anger actually tends to increase and prolong feelings of hostility. Although this finding runs counter to my personal experience and that of many of my patients who have benefited from this practice, there are several additional steps that can be taken to release anger. You can start by recognizing that your anger may be the result of unreasonable or even irrational demands you've made on yourself or someone else, and that by maintaining these demands you are hurting yourself with increased stress. It is therefore in your best interest to release the demands and let go of the anger.

Aerobic exercise

This is another quick-fix method for dissipating anger and opening your nose and sinuses. However, if you're especially enraged about a particular incident or situation, wait at least twenty minutes and take some deep breaths before beginning a strenuous workout. There can be a greater risk of heart attack associated with exercise *immediately* following emotional trauma. Journaling, which I'll discuss in the next section, is also an effective means of releasing anger but not quite as fast as punching and exercise.

DREAMWORK AND JOURNALING

Dreams can play an important role in your healing journey. Serving as symbolic expressions of your inner emotional life, dreams often provide the clues you need to better understand your mental and emotional states, as well as the guidance you may need to heal personal life situations. Dreams can also sometimes reveal how to heal physical disease conditions. This was illustrated in a dream of Alexander the Great recounted in Pliny's

Natural History. One of Alexander's friends, Ptolemaeus, was dying of a poisoned wound, when Alexander dreamed of a dragon holding a plant in its mouth. The dragon said that the plant was the key to curing Ptolemaeus. Upon awakening, Alexander dispatched soldiers to the place he had seen in his dream. They returned with the plant and, as the dream had predicted, Ptolemaeus, as well as many others of Alexander's troops suffering from similar wounds, was cured.

In American society, dreams are often overlooked or ignored, although researchers like Stephen LaBarge, Ph.D., have in recent decades done much to scientifically demonstrate their importance. The two biggest obstacles that prevent us from getting the most benefit from our dreams are that we either do not remember or quickly forget them, or we do not know how to interpret the symbolism and imagery that dreams contain. Dream recall is a skill that anyone can develop with time and practice, however. One of the keys to dreamwork is to commit to focusing attention on your dreams. A deceptively simple way to do this is to tell yourself each night before you fall asleep that when you awaken you will remember what you dreamt during the night. At first you may not experience much success, but regular affirmation of this technique will instruct your unconscious to eventually make your dreams recallable.

As you start to remember your dreams, keep a pad and pencil or a tape recorder by your bed so that you can either write down or verbally record them immediately after you awaken. All of us dream an average of three or four times each night. With practice, many people who make the commitment to record and study their dreams are able to train themselves to spontaneously awaken after each dream cycle to record the gist of their dreams before settling back to sleep until after their next dream stage. Recording your dreams *immediately* after you awaken provides the best results, since dreams are quickly forgotten once you get out of bed and begin your day. Initially, all you may recall are fragments of your dream experience. Don't be discouraged if this is the case. Over time, the regular recording of your dreams will begin to yield more details. In addition, after you have recorded your dreams for a few weeks or months, as you read over your dream diary, you will start to notice how certain symbols and events tend to recur. Pay attention to such common themes: Usually they contain the most important messages that your dreams have for you.

Learning how to interpret the symbolism of your dreams takes time and practice. Certain psychotherapists, especially those with a background in Jungian theory, are skilled in dream interpretation and can help you, and a number of books on the subject can also guide you. Bear in mind, however, that your dreams are highly personal, and although many dream symbols do seem to be common to what Jung called "the collective unconscious," there is no such thing as a standard for dream interpretation that will work for everyone. As the dreamer of your own life, you are ultimately the person best suited to appreciate your dreams and discern their deepest meanings. By taking the time to do so, you can improve your mental and emotional health immeasurably.

Journaling is another simple but very effective way to become more conscious of your mental and emotional life and to help you better express your feelings. The practice of journaling entails keeping a written record of your thoughts, emotions, and any other daily experiences that you would like to better understand. Instead of recording your dreams, you will be keeping a journal of your waking activities. When journaling is done on a regular basis, it usually results in increased self-knowledge, often with insights that are both enlightening and enlivening. In a very real sense, journaling can help you become your own therapist or best friend: Instead of trying to express what you're feeling to someone else, through the process of journaling you tell it to yourself. The result is that your journal becomes your own emotional diary.

Many people who begin the practice of journaling are amazed to discover how the simple act of writing out one's daily experiences can lead to sudden or deeper insights into what they are feeling. Journaling can also help you become better aware of your beliefs, providing you with the opportunity to recognize and change those that may be limiting you. As you journal you will also start to take more control over what you are thinking and feeling, becoming less reactive to your life experiences and more creative in your approaches to dealing with them. Journaling also makes communicating with yourself easier and allows greater clarity, since you are free from judgment or criticism from others. Your journal is for you alone and isn't meant to be shared. Nor do you have to worry about spelling or grammar.

A number of researchers, including James W. Pennebaker, Ph.D., author of the book *Opening Up,* have documented the benefits that journaling can provide by writing about upsetting or traumatic experiences. For people who have difficulty expressing their emotions, particularly those that are judged to be negative, such as anger or fear, journaling can be especially valuable as a tool for self-healing. The results of a recent study measuring the effects of writing about stressful experiences on symptom reduction in patients with mild to moderate asthma and arthritis were published in *JAMA* in April 1999. The subjects in the study were asked to write about the most stressful event of their lives for twenty minutes for three consecutive days. They changed *nothing else* in their treatment regimen. Four months later, researchers found a marked improvement in lung function in the asthmatics and a significant reduction in the severity of disease in the arthritics. This landmark study is a clear demonstration of the therapeutic value of expressing emotions in treating a physical condition. Since most patients with headaches don't have the opportunity to relate their feelings to their physician, writing in a journal or writing unsent letters can be a highly effective self-care technique.

For best results, try to write in your journal around the same time each day. This will help you make journaling a healthy habit. Just before you go to bed can be an ideal time for journaling. You can express the emotions that you've been containing all day and can provide resolution to the day's events prior to going to sleep. Journaling and dreamwork will not only help you to heal mentally and emotionally (and physically), but can also open up new vistas of adventure that can last you a lifetime.

WORK AND PLAY

Do you enjoy your job? Does your work utilize your greatest talents? Is your job fulfilling and challenging? Sadly, for the majority of Americans the answer to these questions is no. Recent studies reveal that an alarmingly high proportion of our society—nearly 70 percent of us—do not experience satisfaction from our jobs. Unfortunately, there is a significant price to be paid for not loving your work, both physiologically and psychologically. For example, in a study conducted by the Massachusetts Department of Health in the late 1980s, it was found that the two greatest risk factors for heart disease lie in one's self-happiness rating and their level of job satisfaction. Low scores in these two areas were shown to be better indicators of the likelihood for developing heart disease than high cholesterol, high blood pressure, obesity, and a sedentary lifestyle. No wonder, then, that in the United States more heart attacks occur on Monday morning around nine o'clock than at any other time of the week.

Your job is a vital aspect of your mental health. If you find yourself working at a job that you do not enjoy, chances are that you continue to do so because of one or more of the following limiting beliefs: *I don't have a choice; I need the money; I'll never be able to make enough money doing what I love; I have no idea what I'd enjoy doing or what my greatest talents are.* By using the techniques outlined in this chapter, especially in the section "Beliefs, Attitudes, Goals, and Affirmations," you can begin to liberate yourself from these unhealthy beliefs. You'll discover that you are not bound to your job for life and you do have the ability to find a job for which you are better suited and that is more fulfilling. Every one of us is blessed with at least one God-given talent, and there is at least one activity that we enjoy doing that we do quite well. *That* is where you need to begin to investigate what your gifts are. Write down your talents as outlined in the goal-setting section above, followed by a list of activities you truly enjoy. Then brainstorm all the possible ways you can think of in which you can earn a living combining your talents with each of the activities you wrote down. List every idea that occurs to you, regardless of how ridiculous it may seem. As you continue to practice this exercise, you will have a much clearer idea of new job options. At the same time, acknowledge that you are seeking a greater level of fulfillment, are willing to change and take a risk, and are committed to begin the exploration that will lead you to work that you love doing. In the process, you may discover that your capabilities are limitless.

Even if you are fortunate to have a job you do enjoy, you may still be prey to another modern day dis-ease, **workaholism.** According to the Economic Policy Institute in Washington, D.C., the majority of Americans are working longer and harder than they used to. Our yearly workload has increased by 158 hours, compared to that of twenty years ago, including longer commuting times and fewer paid holidays and vacation time. That's the equivalent of an extra month's work per year. To counter this tendency, and this is especially important for migraineurs, it is essential that you regularly engage in the counterbalance to work: *play.*

Many of us have unfortunately relegated play to childhood; yet play is a crucial aspect of mental health and is unrivaled as a means of expressing joy, passion, exhilaration, even ecstasy. The word *play* comes from the Middle Dutch *pleyen,* which means "to dance, leap for joy, and rejoice," all activities that suggest a vibrantly healthy mental state. Play has also been defined as any activity in which you lose track of time. Believing that play is not appropriate adult behavior is both limiting and unhealthy.

If your work involves your greatest talents and is something you truly enjoy doing, work and play for you can seem virtually indistinguishable. Even so, to optimize mental health, find at least one other activity to participate in, besides your work, that you can thoroughly enjoy. Such activities include sports, games, dance, and active creative pursuits such as playing a musical instrument, acting, singing, painting, crafts, or gardening. Although many people derive great pleasure from playing cards, chess, and other board games, or stamp or coin collecting, all of these are mental pursuits. To create a healthier balance, select activities that utilize your body, allow you to better express your feelings and creativity, and perhaps even bring you to a greater level of spiritual attunement. Ideally the activity should be something so consuming and absorbing that it requires your total attention, providing a pleasurable escape from your normal tension, stress, and habitual thought patterns. Choose something that instinctively appeals to you and do it on a regular basis, for at least an hour three times a week. Be prepared to make mistakes and look silly. That's part of the risk, and the excitement, of doing something new. The more you commit to and practice whatever activity you choose, the better you'll become at it and the more you'll enjoy the benefits it provides.

We live in a society where work has become the greatest addiction, and the majority of us gauge our self-worth according to our achievements and net worth. For this reason alone the importance of play cannot be overemphasized. All of us, for a short time at least, need to regularly let go of that responsible, mature, working adult part of ourselves to reconnect with our woefully neglected playful "inner child."

SUMMARY

The biggest obstacles each of us must overcome in order to achieve optimal mental and emotional health are our largely unconscious denial and repression of emotional pain, and our limiting thoughts, beliefs, and attitudes, which combined create our unhealthy behaviors. The tools in this chapter will enable you to heighten your awareness, allowing you to consciously transform your life in harmony with your greatest needs and desires. The more you practice the methods outlined here, the more profound the impact you will have on your mental and emotional health, as well as your physical health and your headaches. *You will become more conscious of your behavior and gain the freedom to choose how you wish to think, feel, and behave.* By letting go of your fear of experiencing life more fully (and that includes the fear of making mistakes), you can relax while embracing and accepting all of your thoughts, beliefs, and emotions. This will allow you the joy of realizing your life's goals and the exhilaration of the unimpeded free flow of life-force energy. Remember, only through fully experiencing *both pain and joy* can you truly use your unique gifts and talents to thrive and fulfill your life purpose. And *if you can't feel it, you can't heal it.* This holds true for headaches, arthritis, sinusitis, heart problems, or any other chronic dis-ease. Your underlying emotional pain will be mirrored back to you with the ill health of your body and/or your mind. But so, too, will vitality and happiness reflect a condition of radiant health.

Chapter 6

HEALING YOUR SPIRIT
The Spiritual Health Components
of the Headache Survival Program

What profit does a man receive if he gains the whole world only to lose his soul?
—Matthew 16:26

Components of Optimal Spiritual Health
Experience of unconditional love/absence of fear
- Soul awareness and a personal relationship with God or Spirit
- Trusting your intuition and an openness to change
- Gratitude
- Creating a sacred space on a regular basis through prayer, meditation, walking in nature, observing a Sabbath day, or other rituals
- Sense of purpose
- Being present in every moment

The ultimate outcome of healing ourselves holistically is the recognition that we are truly spiritual beings, and the heightened awareness of the transcendent power known as God or Spirit. By making the commitment to become spiritually healthy, we open ourselves to the underlying life-force energy to which all religions refer, known in holistic medicine as *unconditional love*. Learning to love yourself in body, mind, and spirit is also the simplest and most direct way to learn to love God. To heal yourself spiritually means developing a relationship with Spirit in your own life and attuning yourself to Its guidance in all aspects of your daily existence. By doing so, you will begin to experience a profound reduction in your feelings of fear, and a greater capacity for loving yourself and others unconditionally. You will also become better able to identify your special talents and gifts and use them to fulfill your life's purpose *while fully experiencing the power of the present moment.*

In the deepest sense, all *dis-ease* can be seen as a disconnection between ourselves and Spirit, and a deprivation of love. From that perspective, spiritual health encompasses not only a conscious awareness of the Divine, but also an intimate connection to ourselves, our families, our friends, and our communities. Just as mental health encompasses emotional health, spiritual health embraces social health. You cannot have one without the other. This truth is illustrated in the lives of the world's great spiritual teachers, including Moses, Jesus, Mohammed, Krishna, and Buddha, all of whom remained closely connected to their communities throughout the course of their ministries. Despite the apparent differences in their instructions to us, at their core, their messages are actually the same: *Place God first in all that you do, and love your neighbor as you love yourself.* As you reclaim your spiritual health, you fulfill their intention.

ACCESSING SPIRIT

Every advance in knowledge brings us face to face with the mystery of our own being. —MAX PLANCK, father of quantum physics

You may believe that you are incapable of experiencing Spirit in your life, but that is not the case. *Spirit is present in any moment when we feel profoundly alive.* During these special moments, our predominant emotions are exhilaration and joy. Not surprisingly, most people with migraine or any other chronic illness generally have a lack of joy in their lives. The late Jesuit priest and scientist Teilhard de Chardin described *joy* as "the most infallible sign of the presence of God." Usually these fleeting moments surprise us: Our perception of reality is suddenly free of our normal judgments and concerns. Time seems to slow as we lose ourselves in *pure awareness*. Examples of these moments include experiencing the birth of your child, time spent with your beloved, being present at the death of someone you love, witnessing a sunset, entering "the zone" while playing sports, and being in the presence of inspirational works of art. Such peak experiences can also occur unexpectedly and spontaneously during the course of your normal routine, sparked by something as innocuous as hearing your favorite song on the radio. For most of us, these moments may seem to be accidental occurrences.

The purpose of this chapter is to help make your encounters with Spirit a more frequent and conscious part of your life. As you learn to master the techniques that follow, recognize that Spirit operates in much the same fashion as do subatomic particles: Both can be identified without being directly observed. Most often, and especially at the beginning of your spiritual journey, Spirit will be identified by the traces It leaves behind as It flows through you. With time and attention, each of us can deepen our perception of Spirit in our lives. Among the ways of doing so are *prayer, meditation, gratitude, spiritual practices, reconnecting with nature,* and *working with spiritual counselors.*

ARE WE SPIRITUAL BEINGS? THE NEAR-DEATH EXPERIENCE

Most of us spend our lives deluded by the belief that our traits, habits, and actions are the sum total of who we are. In actuality these characteristic behaviors make up only our conscious personalities, or the sense of self that psychology refers to as the ego. Our ego is the source of our thoughts, judgments, and comparisons, which usually are based on past experience or future concerns. Largely fear-based, the ego diverts our attention from appreciating the reality that exists in the present moment.

We live most of our waking hours in this ego state; yet our true self, the soul (the individualized expression of Spirit), extends well beyond the limits of comprehension of the human intellect.

Letting go of the ego entails a surrender of mind and body that most of us equate with death. The thought of our death can be overpoweringly frightful. However, it is also one of the surest methods for reconnecting with our true spiritual natures. Every experience we have of transcendence and Spirit is also one in which we feel exhilarated and access a dimension of being beyond body and mind. If death is the freeing of our deeper self, or soul, from the physical plane, isn't it possible that it, too, can be an exhilarating experience? Certainly that is the report given by the vast majority of people who have had "near-death experiences." These episodes, also known as NDEs, involve people who were considered clinically dead in emergency or operating rooms, or at the scenes of accidents, and were subsequently resuscitated. In almost every case, these people report experiencing profound feelings of peace and unconditional love, as well as a reluctance to leave the spiritual dimension to return to their bodies. They also report much less fear of death and a greater appreciation for life.

The consistency of the reports of NDEs confirms the observation of many physicians and researchers who have scientifically studied the phenomena of death and dying that the soul remains intact beyond the death of the body. One of the leaders in this field is Elisabeth Kübler-Ross, M.D., who has pioneered this investigation for most of her professional career. After nearly thirty years of scientific research, she has concluded that "death does not exist . . . all that dies is a physical shell housing an immortal spirit." She also describes the time that we spend on earth as but a brief part of our total existence, and teaches that *to live well while we are here means to learn to love*—which is an active recognition, engagement, and appreciation of Spirit in ourselves and others. In one of her studies of over two hundred people who had experienced a near-death experience, almost all reported that they went before God and were asked the question

"How have you expanded your ability to give and receive love while you were down there?"

Whether or not you choose to believe the data being gathered in the fields of thanatology and NDE, there is mounting evidence strongly suggesting the existence of Spirit beyond the realms of mind and body. Choosing to believe this theory can heighten your creativity, enhance your healing capacity, free you to realize your life's purpose, diminish the level of fear in your life, and release the self-imposed limitations of past traumas. By becoming more aware of your soul—that part of yourself that does not die—you will be better able to take risks and pursue the dreams of your life.

6. Prayer

The most common form of spiritual exercise engaged in by most Americans is prayer. Nearly 90 percent of us pray, and 70 percent of us believe that prayer can lead to physical, emotional, or spiritual healing. Most people who pray have a greater sense of well-being than those who don't, and, when polled, the majority of people who pray say that through prayer they experience a sense of peace, receive answers to life issues, and have even felt divinely inspired or "led by God" to perform some specific action. Interestingly, people who experience a "sense of the Divine" during prayer also score the highest on ratings of general well-being and satisfaction with their lives.

In recent years, a great deal of scientific study has focused on the beneficial effects of prayer. Among the studies is one by the National Institute of Mental Health in 1994, which examined nearly three thousand North Carolinians and found that those who attended church weekly had 29 percent less risk of alcoholism than those who attended less frequently. In the same study, the risk of alcoholism decreased by 42 percent among those who prayed and read the Bible regularly. Another NIMH study conducted in the same year found that frequent churchgoers also had lower rates of depression and other mental problems.

An examination of 212 medical studies examining the relationship between religious beliefs and health by Dale Matthews, M.D., associate professor of medicine at Georgetown University, found that 75 percent of the studies showed health benefits for those patients with "religious commitments." Among patients with hypertension, regular prayer reduced blood pressure in 50 percent of all cases.

Among the pioneers in the study of the physiological effects of prayer and meditation is Herbert Benson, M.D., a Harvard cardiologist. In 1968, Benson began studying people who regularly practiced transcendental meditation (TM). The subjects meditated by focusing on a mantra, such as *Om,* that had no apparent meaning to its user. Benson discovered that repetition of the mantra resulted in a lower metabolic rate, slower heart rate, lower blood pressure, and slower breathing. He dubbed this physiological effect the *relaxation response* (RR). Benson then turned his attention to Christians and Jews who prayed instead of meditating, instructing them to repeat religious phrases such as the first line of the Lord's Prayer, "Hail Mary, full of grace," "The Lord is my shepherd," or "Shalom." He found that the phrases all produced the same relaxation response that is triggered by meditation, and that the degree of physiological benefit is determined by the degree of faith on the part of the person praying.

Since 1988, Benson and psychologist Jared Klass have been conducting a series of programs at the Mind/Body Medical Institute at New England Deaconess Hospital, inviting priests, rabbis, and ministers to investigate the spiritual and health implications of prayer. In their studies, a psychological scale developed by Benson and Klass for measuring spirituality is employed. People scoring high in spirituality—defined by Benson as a feeling that "there is more than just you" and as not necessarily religious—score higher in psychological health. They also:

• were less likely to get sick, and were better able to cope if they did

- had fewer stress-related symptoms
- gained the most from meditation training
- showed the greatest rise on a life-purpose index
- exhibited the sharpest drop in pain

To begin the practice of prayer, start with any prayer you are comfortable with or recall from your religious training as a child. You can also use a favorite psalm or passage from the Bible or prayer book you find especially meaningful. In addition, you can engage in personal prayer, talking to God as if you were speaking to your best friend. State your need or concern and ask for God's help. (It is more effective to pray for the peace that would result from having what you desire, than pray for the specific things themselves.)

In an experiment performed by the Spindrift organization in Lansdale, Pennsylvania, the effectiveness of directed and nondirected prayer was tested. Those practicing directed prayer had a specific goal, image, or outcome in mind, while nondirected prayer is an open-ended approach in which no specific outcome is held in mind. The practitioner of nondirected prayer does not attempt "to tell the universe what to do." The results proved conclusively that chances are much greater for attaining the desired outcome when one prays for "what's best"—"Thy will be done." Whichever form of prayer you choose, try to establish a regular routine and repeat your prayer morning and night.

Gratitude

I include *gratitude* and *prayer* together as number 6 in my list of the *essential 8 for optimal health.* Most religious traditions prescribe specific prayers or grace before meals as a way of thanking God for our food and sustenance. As with other spiritual practices, there is something to be gained from these rituals or they wouldn't have survived for thousands of years. A sense of gratitude for all the other areas of our lives can elicit similar life-enhancing benefits.

Gratitude has been called the "Great Attitude." Although most of us tend to take our lives for granted, they are in fact a gift, and every day that we are alive each of us receives many blessings. Even times of pain and fear, such as a particularly severe headache, can be seen as opportunities for growth for which we can be grateful. A migraine attack can at times be so terrifying that the migraineur feels as if he or she is dying or would like to die. Although this usually results in a greater level of general anxiety, it is possible for this individual to develop a far greater appreciation of life. By committing ourselves to becoming more aware of our blessings, we strengthen our connection with Spirit and are able to better recognize the wisdom and intelligence that underlie all of creation.

Once we allow ourselves to appreciate the lessons presented during times of struggle or life crises, the brunt of the pain subsides and a state of inner peace follows. This is especially true of most chronic diseases, which can be seen as external reflections of inner (emotional and/or spiritual) pain. Typically, when people choose to consciously focus on the positives in their lives and express gratitude for them, more positive things start to happen. For instance, while you're learning to live with your headaches, suppose you spent time each day focusing on the blessings and the many pleasures your body has provided you with in the past along with the multitude of basic functions for which it still serves you well. These include the ability to enjoy breathing, eating, drinking, digesting, eliminating, exercising, and making love. Although you have a chronic physical problem, which at times is incapacitating, you've still retained the capacity to choose your beliefs and attitudes, as well as to experience, express, and accept all of your feelings. In addition, this physical disability can serve as a powerful catalyst for becoming better acquainted with your soul and Spirit. You may have never recognized the spiritual being that you truly are, or your purpose for being here, had you not been blessed with migraine. This may sound unreasonable or even irrational to you, but it was certainly helpful to me in curing my chronic sinusitis. For many years I suffered and felt as if I were cursed. I angrily asked of

God, "Why me? What have I done to deserve this misery?" Yet now I can clearly see how this physical pain has so enriched my life. It's taught me how to give and receive love—to nurture my body, home and work environments, mind, emotional body, intimate relationships, and my soul. This is the essence of the work I came here to do, and it has become my full-time job. I call it training to thrive, and at fifty-four, I'm healthier and more fit physically, mentally, and spiritually than I've ever been. Who knows what my life would have been like had I not been blessed with sinusitis, or yours without headaches?

Gratitude can produce powerful feelings of joy and self-acceptance, and is an attitude that anyone can choose to have, just as you can choose to see the glass half full or half empty. By focusing on what you do have instead of what you lack, you feel a sense of abundance that makes your problems seem much less acute, and you are better able to let go of negative thoughts and attitudes. This usually isn't easy to do, especially if you are feeling a great deal of fear or anger. But if you make the effort to release these painful emotions and *choose the attitude of gratitude,* even for a moment, wonderful things can happen.

Like any habit, that of recognizing and acknowledging the gifts in your life requires practice. One simple way to begin feeling grateful is the following visualization taught by Rabbi Mordecai Twerski, the spiritual leader of Denver's Hasidic community. As soon as you wake up each morning, before you get out of bed, close your eyes and picture a person, scene, or situation that made you happy to be alive and for which you are still grateful. You never would have had that experience if you weren't alive, and by allowing yourself to reexperience it, you open yourself up to the awareness that something equally wonderful can happen today. Create the habit of practicing this visualization each morning upon awakening and you will soon instill in yourself a new attitude of anticipation and appreciation for the day ahead.

Another way to cultivate feelings of gratitude is by making a *gratitude list.* This exercise is best performed before going to bed, as a way to detach yourself from any concerns or problems you may have in order to appreciate the gifts and lessons that came your way during the day. Some people prefer to write out their list; others simply close their eyes and mentally review their day, making themselves aware of all the things that happened for which they feel grateful. Either way works well. Complete the exercise by praying silently, giving thanks for all that you experienced and learned that day.

By making gratitude a regular part of your daily experience, you set the stage for living more deeply connected to Spirit. In the process, your life will be transformed into an increasingly joyous adventure.

MEDITATION

In the West, meditation has primarily been studied for its mental, emotional, and physiological benefits, while in the East it has primarily been used for thousands of years to still the mind in order to heighten awareness and contact soul and Spirit. During meditation, practitioners enter into a neutral emotional state, becoming a witness to their passing thoughts and feelings as they move into a state of heightened attention that can ultimately result in pure awareness.

As with prayer, there are many ways to meditate. Meditation can be performed while sitting or in a supine position, or while on the move—walking, jogging, and even during sports. What all forms of meditation have in common is a focusing on the breath and an emptying of the mind of thought. With regular practice, meditators typically report increased feelings of calm and peace, improved mental functioning and enhanced powers of concentration, and a deeper connection to Spirit, which is often perceived as a quiet, inner voice guiding them in their actions. Other reported benefits include increased equanimity toward, and detachment from, life events; increased energy and joy; feelings of bliss and ecstasy; and increased dream recall.

It is best to learn meditation under the guidance of a qualified instructor, but a variety of books and audiotapes are also available on the subject. The simplest method of meditation is to sit in a quiet place, resting comfortably in a chair, with your spine erect and your feet flat on the floor. Close your eyes and begin focusing on your breathing, keeping your awareness on each inhalation and exhalation. The practice is done using belly or abdominal breathing (see page 81). To improve your concentration, you may wish to silently repeat the word *in* as you inhale, and *out* as you exhale. Or you can repeat a word or mantra, such as *love, peace, God, Om,* or *Hu* (both latter terms are names for the Divine). Allow your thoughts to come and go without lingering on them, as if your awareness were a running stream and your thoughts were simply leaves floating by. At first you may feel deluged with thoughts. Each time you find yourself distracted, simply bring your attention back to your breathing. Eventually you may notice longer periods of silence between each thought. It may take months to quiet your mind to this extent, but with consistent practice your meditation *will* become deeper and easier. Try to sit for at least ten minutes once or twice a day, gradually working up to two half-hour sessions per day. It's important to keep your practice regular and consistent, but don't force things. If you find yourself too distracted or pressed for time, end your session until next time instead of sitting restlessly.

Walking meditation is another form of meditation that in recent years has been popularized by the Buddhist monk Thich Nhat Hanh. This means of meditation is often suited for active people who find it difficult to sit still. The goal is to focus your attention in the present by focusing on each step you take in tandem with your breathing. To enhance your experience, you can mentally repeat *With each step I take I am fully present to my surroundings.* Over time, as you practice this form of meditation, don't be surprised if you find it becomes more difficult to hurry. The more you focus on the present, the less consequence time has as you discover how profound even a simple act such as walking can be.

INTUITION

As you progress in your healing journey, eventually you will find yourself being guided by your intuition, which is often experienced as an "inner nudge" or a "still, quiet voice" speaking from within. If you are not already aware of your intuitive messages, most likely it is because your intuition is having a tough time competing for your attention. Most of the inner messages you hear come from your ego and tend to be loud, self-centered, and fear-based. Intuitive messages, by contrast, come from the heart and are usually more subtle, compassionate, energizing, and enlivening.

In order to develop your sense of intuition, you will need to slow down, eliminate distractions, and do a lot less talking. The methods provided in this chapter can help you to do so. Slow, relaxing walks are another helpful way to make contact with this inner guidance. The next step is learning to recognize when your intuition is truly speaking to you, and when it is not. Learning to discern the difference requires practice. One useful method for determining if the "voice" you hear is indeed your intuition is to notice how it feels. Often intuitive messages occur accompanied by feelings of excitement or an unequivocal sense that acting upon them is "the right thing to do." People who haven't learned to trust their intuition often experience doubts or fears immediately following such feelings. "How can I be sure this is true?" "What if I'm wrong?" These and similar questions can quickly quash your inner guidance if you haven't learned to trust it.

To help you know if the messages you receive are in your best interest, experiment with the following exercise. Out loud, tell yourself something that you know to be true. As you do so, notice how you feel. Now state aloud something you know to be false. Again notice how you feel. Usually people practicing this exercise experience feelings of discomfort, confusion, even pain, in their bodies when they make the false statement, whereas they feel in alignment with the statement that is true. (Often the sensations occur in the area of the solar plexus, with false statements provoking queasy feelings or tension.)

Allowing yourself to be guided by your intuition is ultimately an act of faith. At first, learning to trust and act on the intuitive messages you receive will involve risk. The more trust you bring to your practice, however, the easier it will be to take action. Realize, too, that sometimes the results of following your intuition may be painful. Such times are not necessarily mistakes. They can be seen as lessons teaching you how to listen more effectively. Or they may be necessary to facilitate your growth and help you to better understand the higher purpose toward which Spirit is guiding you.

SPIRITUAL COUNSELORS

Due to the many uncertainties that can be part of the spiritual journey, you may consider working with a spiritual counselor, especially if you haven't been in the habit of listening to your intuition or need help in "tuning in" to Spirit. Just as you would visit a doctor to heal your physical body, or a psychotherapist to heal mental and emotional issues, spiritual counselors can help connect you to your spiritual core. The most common resources for spiritual counseling are priests, rabbis, ministers, and other clergy. Spiritual psychotherapists, medical intuitives, clairvoyants, and spiritual healers or shamans can also be of great assistance. What these healers have in common is an ability to see beyond the boundaries of the five senses. Their services may include helping you to identify your life purpose, pointing out opportunities for your spiritual growth, or scanning your body's bio-energy field to diagnose the underlying cause of a particular health condition. Their primary value, however, lies in the assistance they can provide in helping you appreciate the meaning and lessons of your daily life, especially those that are most painful.

Because of the lack of certification in these areas, to find a spiritual counselor, you may need to rely on references from people you trust, experience some trial and error, and call upon your own intuition. Keep an open mind and see how you respond to the information provided. Some of these counselors are truly gifted and can provide you with information that can be a catalyst for transforming your life.

SPIRITUAL PRACTICES

Most of us have some sort of spiritual orientation, even if it is no more than what we received in childhood. Yet, we often fail to realize how much some of these practices can contribute to our health. The ritual observance of *Sabbath,* for instance, can be an enormously healing experience, as it restores the sacred rhythm between work and rest. We're so busy *doing* in our society that we've forgotten how to just *be* and appreciate the delight of simply being alive. The Sabbath day is also a particularly good time to practice gratitude as you contemplate the blessings you share with those you love. Studies also reveal that those who regularly observe a weekly holy day tend to score higher in areas of optimism, stress management, and general well-being.

Fasting is another spiritual practice that is also healing. Not only can fasting have a cleansing effect upon the body, eliminating toxins while giving the organs of digestion and assimilation a rest, it can also elicit a heightened feeling of spirituality and result in the healing of old emotional wounds. In his book *Live Better Longer,* Joseph Dispenza, director of the Parcells Center in Santa Fe, New Mexico, points out that fasting can purge the emotional body of old, toxic feelings, facilitate the release of psychological patterns that no longer work for you, and "open your mind and heart to new emotional, psychological, and spiritual sustenance." (The Parcells Center is based on the work of Dr. Hazel Parcells, a scientist and naturopathic physician who, at forty-one, cured herself of terminal tuberculosis using fasts and other natural methods. She then went on to live a life of vibrant, robust health until she died peacefully in her sleep at age 106.)

If you are new to fasting, try a twenty-four-hour fast, selecting a day when work and other responsibilities are limited and you won't be too active. Plan for some quiet time alone and, during the final two hours of the fast, drink six to eight glasses of water to help cleanse your body of toxins.

Gabriel Cousens, M.D., at his Tree of Life Rejuvenation Center in Patagonia, Arizona, has had great success in treating a variety of diseases, including asthma, arthritis, diabetes, and alcoholism, with fasting and meditation.

The potential that spiritual practices have to heal is illustrated in the case of one of my friend and colleague Dr. Bob Anderson's patients, a sixty-four-year-old woman named Lois, who underwent the surgical removal of a very large, aggressive ovarian cancer. The procedure left her with a colostomy, and part of the original tumor was not removable, leaving hundreds of small metastases throughout her abdominal cavity. On Dr. Anderson's insistence, Lois agreed to consult with an oncologist, only to promptly reject his recommendation of chemotherapy despite the fact that remnants of her tumor remained in her pelvis and abdomen. She was convinced that her condition would be cured by her own body with God's help, and returned to Dr. Anderson to aid her in getting well. Although she undertook many initiatives, central to her program was her faith in the power of prayer and God. Each day she meditated for up to an hour and prayed numerous times.

Four months later Lois was finally able to persuade her surgeon to remove the colostomy to restore her internal bowel function. During the course of a long and tedious surgery, hundreds of small, metastasized tumors appeared as before. Seven of them were biopsied. Three days later, the pathology report showed that their cancerous characteristics were gone. Lois fully recovered and resumed an active life focused around the activities she enjoyed and her continued prayers to God. Two years later, an operation to repair an abdominal hernia revealed that her abdomen and pelvis were completely normal, with no residual cancer anywhere. Although he has no way of proving it, Dr. Anderson remains convinced that Lois's daily prayers and meditations were somehow central to her recovery.

Finding Spirit in Nature

Nowhere is the creative power of Spirit more visible than in nature. It is here that we most directly experience life's four elemental forms of energy: earth, water, fire, and air. Earth is matter in its deepest form; water represents the receptive yielding principle; fire is the transformational energy that causes matter to change form; and air is the resultant blend of these other three elements into a subtler vibration of life-force energy. In our bodies, earth is cellular matter, water is blood and circulation, fire is metabolism and energy production, and air is oxygen, the nutrient most essential for our sustenance. By regularly exposing yourself to nature's four elements—ideally on a daily basis—you will expand your awareness of how each of them is uniquely embodied within you and more fully appreciate the healing power of nature. What follows are ways for you to do so.

Earth.

Spend as much time as possible outdoors in close contact with the earth. Walking is a wonderful way to do this, as are outdoor sports, bike rides in a park, and gardening. When you can, also visit the beach, woods, and mountains, and take time to notice the beauty surrounding you. The more time you spend immersed in nature, the more aware you will become of life's natural rhythms and the ways the earth retains and radiates energy.

As a society, we need to recognize that cities and other industrialized areas are in fact unnatural and can keep us from living a life of balance. Making the effort to spend time in nature can go a long way to restoring that balance while deepening your connection with Spirit at the same time.

Water.

One of the most visible forms of Spirit in nature is the flow of water as it follows the contours of the earth. Water is a receptive form of energy and is affected by the forces acting upon it. Rivers flow, for example, due to the gravitational pull caused by the gradient of the landscape. The action of water tumbling over rocks also releases a more subtle energy in the form of negative ions, which can contribute to feelings of well-being. Swimming in the ocean, lakes, or rivers provides invaluable exposure to this special form of energy. Soaking in a mineral hot spring can also provide therapeutic benefits for a variety of ailments, and can be one of life's great pleasures.

A healthy routine that anyone can adopt is bathing in warm water at least once a day. For added benefit, practice belly breathing while you enjoy a soak in the tub. This is a very effective way to connect with your body's bioenergy field, and can help heal mental and emotional upset.

Fire.

Throughout the Bible and other sacred scriptures, the dominant symbols of the divine essence in human beings is fire and light, such as the tale of Moses speaking to God in the burning bush, or the transfiguration of Jesus on the mountaintop before his closest apostles. Candlelight is also common as a tool for spiritual focus in most religions. Anyone who has experienced the pleasures of an open campfire can attest to the healing properties of fire. According to Leonard Orr, the founder of Rebirthing, spending time before an open fire, including a fireplace, cleanses the bioenergy field of negative energies and can be a powerful aid in curing physical disease. Orr recommends spending a few hours each day before fire for people who want to experience such benefits.

Fire is also an important component of the vision quests employed by Native Americans as a means of connecting to Spirit and discerning their life purpose. The ultimate source of fire energy is the sun, which provides healing and creative energy that directly or indirectly gives life to all living organisms. Regular exposure to sunlight has been linked to a variety of mental and emotional benefits, while depression, anxiety, and other mental dis-ease can occur when we are deprived of the sun's healing rays (e.g., seasonal affective disorder, or SAD). Time spent daily in the sun is a very healthy practice as long as appropriate precautions are taken, including sunscreen, hats, and long sleeves and pants when needed.

Air.

Of the four elements, air is perhaps the closest expression of Spirit, so much so that the ancient Greeks equated Spirit (*pneuma*) with the wind. The most potent method of imbuing yourself with the life-force energy of air is through meditation and other forms of conscious breathing. A daily practice of these methods can significantly energize you, open you up to new levels of creativity and productivity, and make you more aware of Spirit's guidance and power flowing through you.

SOCIAL HEALTH

No man is an island. —JOHN DONNE

COMPONENTS OF OPTIMAL SOCIAL HEALTH

Intimacy with a spouse, partner, relative, or close friend
- Effective communication
- Forgiveness
- Touch and/or physical intimacy on a daily basis
- Sense of belonging to a support group or community
- Selflessness and altruism

Our relationship with others is the crucible that most determines how spiritually healthy we are. Optimal *social health* consists of a strong positive connection to others in community and family, and intimacy with one or more people. It is often much easier to feel our connection with Spirit during moments of solitude than it is to express that connection through our interactions with others. At the same time, our relationships offer us the greatest opportunities for spiritual growth and for learning how to receive and impart unconditional love. *True spiritual health is a balance between the autonomy of the self and intimacy with others.*

The importance of social relationships, love, and intimacy with respect to health is documented in a growing number of studies demonstrating the benefits of the diversity and depth of connection to community, family, and spouse. Lack of healthy social relationships is a common denominator among patients with heart disease, particularly when accompanied by feelings of hostility and a sense of isolation. Conversely, the longevity of terminal cancer patients with long-term survival rates has been attributed to a relatively high degree of social involvement. One of the most convincing studies highlighting the importance of community showed that Hispanics, despite poverty, lack of health insurance, and poor access to medical care, are surprisingly less likely than whites to die of major chronic diseases, including all forms of cancer, heart disease, and respiratory ailments. Further, with the exception of diabetes, liver disease, and homicide, their overall health outlook is significantly better than that for whites. Some health experts, including former surgeon general Antonia Coello Novello, the first Latina to serve in that post, postulate that the reason for this stems from Hispanic culture, which promotes strong family values and frowns on health risks such as drinking and smoking. Based on a growing number of relationship studies, researchers have concluded that *social isolation is statistically just as dangerous as smoking, high blood pressure, high cholesterol, obesity, or lack of exercise.*

The primary opportunities available to each of us for improving our social health include marriage, committed relationships, parenting, forgiveness, friendships, selfless acts and altruism, and support groups.

7. Intimacy—Communication, Recreation, Touch

COMMITTED RELATIONSHIPS AND MARRIAGE

Healthy committed relationships are probably the most effective and direct method of experiencing intimacy and unconditional love, in addition to promoting physical, emotional, and especially spiritual well-being. The model for all committed relationships is marriage, usually the most challenging as well as the most rewarding of all interpersonal relationships. It is potentially our most powerful spiritual practice. If humanity's fundamental moral principle is "Love thy neighbor as thyself," its practice begins not with the person living next door, but with the neighbor with whom we share our bed.

Regardless of who your partner may be or how long you have been involved with him or her, the key to all committed relationships is **intimacy.** Think of intimacy as *into-me-see.* As you develop the skills for seeing into—and learning to appreciate—yourself, you have the opportunity to also "see into" your partner and allow your partner to see into you. Once a commitment is made, the relationship becomes greater than the sum of its parts, allowing both partners to flourish and realize their full potential as human beings. The transformation that can occur in marriage and other committed relationships is primarily a result of letting go of judgment. As you do so, you will realize that in giving more to the relationship you are ultimately giving to yourself. Studies have shown that you may otherwise be contributing to making yourself and your partner sick. Marital conflict lowers immune function, especially in women, according to researchers at Ohio State University.

Hallmarks of a healthy committed relationship include *effective communication, recreation,* and *touch.* Good communication encompasses the creation of a shared vision, attentive listening to each other, and the freedom to make requests so that both partners can better ensure that their needs are met. Regular intervals of fun and recreation together with daily doses of physical intimacy and touch provide the glue for most thriving relationships. If you are interested in making a deeper commitment to your relationship, you might also consider working with a good marriage counselor or other relationship teacher.

Shared vision.

A vision that you share with your partner is a way of defining your mutual goals and focusing your energy on their attainment. Lack of a vision can cause your relationship to lose direction or become stagnant. One simple but effective way to create a shared vision with your spouse or partner is to take time to individually list your relationship goals (keep them positive, short, descriptive, specific), prioritizing them in numerical order. Then begin combining lists, starting with the goals having the highest value and alternating between the two lists to form a composite vision you and your partner are both comfortable with. The resulting "mutual relationship vision" can help keep you and your partner working together toward your common goals while reducing conflict and enhancing your relationship.

Attentive listening.

Most of us are poor listeners: We *hear* what is being said, but we don't always *listen* to it. This is because hearing can be unconscious, while listening requires conscious effort. Since communication is the foundation of any relationship, and listening is a critical aspect of effective communication, it is important to get in the habit of consciously paying attention to what your partner tells you *without responding immediately.* The practice of listening can greatly enhance both intimacy and autonomy. This type of listening can be practiced as a "listening exercise." Schedule an uninterrupted forty-minute block of time in which both you and your partner speak for twenty minutes while the other person listens *without responding.* Talk only about yourself and how you're feeling, without blaming or talking about your relationship issues. There is no discussion following the exercise.

Attentive listening makes it possible for both partners to be able to talk freely and express thoughts and feelings without worrying about judgment or criticism. Focusing on what your partner is saying requires you to empty your mind of your own thoughts and concerns as you listen, thereby minimizing negative reactions. This exercise allows for a balance between intimacy and autonomy, a critical component of healthy relationships. Cultivating the habit of attentive listening will help you and your partner create a safe environment for expressing your feelings, allowing you to be more vulnerable and open with each other, which is extremely valuable for building trust, understanding, and deeper, even exhilarating, feelings of intimacy.

Requests.

By committing to another person, you enter into a relationship in which you have promised to give and receive love. But since each of us is different, what feels like love to one person may not even be noticed by another. Most of us attempt to love our partners in ways that feel like love to *us,* and are surprised when they do not react as we would. A good method for eliminating this problem is simply to tell each other what feels good to you and what you want.

It can be quite a revelation when someone you thought you knew well tells you what they really *need* from you. We often expect our partners to be able to read our minds, but we really can't know what each other wants unless we are told. Refrain from general statements such as "Love me" or "Be nice to me." Making specific requests like "I would like you to buy me flowers once a week" or "I would like you to cook dinner once a week" will significantly improve the likelihood that you will get what you need. When you do, be sure to thank your partner for complying with your request. This is extremely important, since your request is usually not an easy or natural thing for your partner to do. Otherwise you probably wouldn't have had to ask for it in the first place.

Having fun together.

Life's daily pressures and responsibilities make it difficult to remember to have fun. For many couples, the glue that reinforces their relationship is the memory of the enjoyment they shared during their courtship and early years together. Setting aside time that you and your partner can spend in recreation together is an important way to *re-create* the joy and spontaneity that first brought you together. To rekindle some of that excitement and minimize the risk of boring routines, it helps to schedule fun activities together on a regular basis. Plan at least half a day each week to spend together away from home, taking turns each time to choose your activity. Getting out of the house, alone together, can help you focus attention on each other. Although this is more difficult to do if you have young children, it is still possible to plan an exciting evening at home after they go to bed. Choose something neither of you has tried before to add another dimension of adventure to your play, and, if you can manage it, plan several weekends per year out of town. This can be especially rewarding if a real vacation isn't feasible. Having fun regularly with the person you love is refreshing and invigorating, and can help ensure that your relationship remains healthy and fulfilling.

TOUCH

Touch is not only one of our most effective healing modalities, it might well be the most powerful and direct means of conveying love. The lack of touch and physical affection is being recognized as a contributing factor in causing asthma, while massage has been shown to improve pulmonary function in children with asthma. According to Saul Schanberg, M.D., Ph.D., a professor of pharmacology and biological chemistry at Duke University, "Humans need to touch and be touched, just as we need food and water." His research and that of other experts were cited in *Hands-on Healing,* edited by John Feltman.

- In a study involving forty premature infants, half of them were gently stroked for forty-five minutes a day; the other twenty were not. Although all were fed the same amount of calories, after ten days, the touched babies weighed in 47 percent heavier than the unstimulated group. The stroked babies were also more active, more alert, and more responsive to social stimulation.
- When a person's wrist is gently held by someone else, the heartbeat slows and blood pressure declines.
- Children and adolescents hospitalized for psychiatric problems show remarkable reductions in anxiety levels and positive changes in attitude when they receive a brief daily back rub.
- The arteries of rabbits fed a high-cholesterol diet and petted regularly had 60 percent less blockage than did the arteries of unpetted but similarly fed rabbits.
- Rats that were handled for fifteen minutes a day during the first three weeks of their lives showed dramatically less cell deterioration and memory loss as they grew old, compared with nonhandled rats.

In a study published in July 2000, Fijian women were found to have the lowest incidence of breast cancer of any country in the world. This was attributed to the practice of breast massage, which all Fijian girls are taught as they reach childbearing age.

Yet in spite of the mounting evidence and healthy reasons to touch and be touched by other human beings (and from the Fijian study, even by ourselves), Americans indulge very little in this simple pleasure. One study in the 1960s noted the number of touches exchanged by pairs of people sitting in coffee shops around the world. In San Juan, Puerto Rico, people touched 180 times an hour; in Paris, France, 110 times an hour; in Gainesville, Florida, 2 times an hour; and in London, England, the pairs never touched. The implications and possible causes of this phenomenon would entail a lengthy discussion, although I am sure the puritanical legacy of associating touch with sex has had a profound effect on American attitudes. William E. Whitehead, Ph.D., an associate professor of medical psychology at the Johns Hopkins University School of Medicine, believes that a significant part of the blame lies with the father of modern-day psychology, Sigmund Freud. "Freud encouraged austerity in dealing with children. And parents bought into that behavior," says Dr. Whitehead. People who aren't cuddled a lot as kids, he adds, tend to develop into nontouching adults. The cycle then repeats itself, generation after generation.

As an osteopathic physician, I learned very early in my medical training about the therapeutic value of the "laying on of hands." Although almost all of our courses and textbooks were the same as those used to train allopathic medical medical doctors (M.D.s), we were also taught a holistic approach to health care that included osteopathic manipulative therapy. Soft-tissue stretching (somewhat similar to massage) and adjustments or corrections in the position of the spine and other body parts (similar to chiropractic adjustments) are part of this therapy. It has taken me a while to realize that patients responded well to this treatment not only because of the prescribed techniques, but also because of the healing potential of the touch itself. It is now apparent that touch is helpful in treating headaches (especially Healing and Therapeutic Touch) as well as most other chronic conditions. There are a number of therapies in which touch is the primary healing ingredient. They include acupressure, chiropractic, craniosacral therapy, healing touch, Hellerwork, various types of massage, physical therapy, reflexology, Rolfing, therapeutic touch, and the Trager approach. If you are interested in experiencing a hands-on healing technique, I suggest trying a practitioner of one of these therapies. And if you're not so inclined, it isn't necessary to visit a professional practitioner to enjoy the benefits of touch. In the study demonstrating the benefits of massage on children with asthma, it was the parents who performed the massage. I don't think most of us require a great deal of instruction on hugging or how to administer a loving touch. *Physical intimacy, including affection, strokes, and hugs, are a cornerstone of healthy relationships.*

Touching with love need not be sexual, nor must it be given or received from another person to be beneficial. Animals are perfectly fine sources of tactile comfort, says Alan M. Beck, Sc.D., director of the Center for the Interaction of Animals and Society at the University of Pennsylvania. Numerous studies, he adds, "definitely show that petting an animal can lower one's blood pressure." Other doctors suggest that there are health benefits to be had even from cuddling inanimate objects—teddy bears, for instance. If you have neither a pet nor a favorite stuffed animal, my prescription for helping to maintain your social health is to get several hugs daily!

There is no question that we have become too distant from one another. At a time when there are more of us than ever before (280 million), many holistic physicians and health care practitioners believe that loneliness may be Americans' greatest health risk. The recent trend toward more touching is our culture's attempt to restore a sense of wholeness and balance, and return to the norms and values of preindustrialized society. Most primitive cultures are very touch oriented. I have lived with one such native group in which touch is the traditional primary mode of healing. These people believe that their healers have a gift bestowed by God, and that the healing energy that flows through the healer to the patient is God's love. Whatever its source, the healer's touch works quite well for a variety of ailments. By our standards these high-touch people might be considered primitive or underdeveloped, but they are clearly much healthier than most Americans in body, mind, and spirit.

SEX

Of all the major world religions, the Judeo-Christian tradition is the only one that does not commonly recognize the potential that sexual intercourse has as a pathway to Spirit. Other religions, including Hinduism, Buddhism, Islam, and Taoism, as well as the spiritual traditions of Africa and the Amerindians, freely acknowledge that sex, properly entered into, can be a powerful spiritual experience capable of transforming consciousness and enhancing physical and emotional health. In the West, perhaps the most well-known of these teachings on sex is *tantra*. This is an ancient system of sexual and sensual techniques for consciously controlling the mind, increasing life-force energy, and tapping into Spirit. Tantra's erotic practices include specific positions, breath, and visualization to heighten sexual energy and move it upward along the spine in order to create rapturous waves of blissful energy that can ultimately lead to enlightenment. Many mystic writings, such as the verse of the Sufi poet-saint Rumi, also refer to the Divine using the language of sex and romantic love, often equating God with the Beloved while yearning to experience union with the Absolute.

To experience sex from this exalted perspective requires expanding your focus beyond physical gratification and genital orgasm, into an experience of yourself and your spouse or lover as expressions of Spirit-in-the-flesh. Adopting this attitude leaves you extremely vulnerable and simultaneously in touch with your own divine power. Lovemaking in this state is free of the machinations of ego and proceeds slowly, gently, and consciously, ensuring that the needs of both partners are always met before moving on to the next cycle of pleasure and awareness. Couples who master this approach are able to remain in a state of heightened excitation for several hours, prolong and intensify orgasm, and experience total-body orgasms. Among the experiences they report are a continuous flow of energy throughout their bodies, a joined climax of body and soul, the sensation of being united with the cosmos, and, afterward, being refreshed and revitalized. The primary goal of "spiritual sex" isn't prolonged orgasm, however, but an experience of being more deeply connected with the person you love and, through that connectedness, an awareness of your integral role within the whole of creation. Not everyone will feel the need to master, or even explore, a tantric approach to sex, yet all of us can benefit from more conscious lovemaking. Of all the spiritual practices, it is certainly the most pleasurable and potentially the most intimacy-enhancing. (To learn more about the tantric approach to sex, see *The Art of Sexual Ecstasy* by Margo Anand.)

PARENTING

Parenting is easily one of life's most enriching experiences and, at the same time, one of our most challenging jobs. Through their children, parents have the opportunity to reconnect with play, to feel more in touch with their own "inner child," to experience selflessness, and to learn how to love unconditionally. Those of us who are parents are also provided with a wonderful forum for practicing forgiveness, trust, acceptance of ourselves and others, self-awareness, and, most of all, patience (as any parent of a teenager well knows). Perhaps the greatest human expression of love is that of parents for their children.

Unfortunately, in our society parenting isn't always consciously approached. If you are already a parent, however, it is not too late to meet your parental obligations more consciously than you may currently be doing. One useful guideline is to regularly ask yourself: *Will this [action, response, activity, demand] of mine help my child's self-esteem?* The same principle holds true in parenting as it does in marriage: *To love another is to help that person better love him- or herself.* This commitment will not only affect your child's happiness in the present but will significantly impact his or her future health. In the landmark Harvard Mastery of Stress Study, college students rated their parents on their level of parental caring. Thirty-five years later, 87 percent of those who rated both parents low on parental love suffered from a chronic illness, whereas only 25 percent of those who rated both parents high in caring had a disease.

In the field of family therapy, the family is usually seen as a "system." This view holds that if a family member's behavior is harmful to himself or others, the problem and the solution lie not only within the individual but within the entire family system. This perspective encourages parents to examine their roles and the responsibility they share with their child for his or her problem. Often, a child's crisis serves as a mirror reflecting an imbalance in his or her individual system as well as in the family system as a whole. One of the significant advantages of family therapy is that change often occurs more rapidly than in individual psychotherapy. In much the same way that holistic medicine treats the entire person, not simply physical symptoms, the family-systems approach recognizes the need for family therapy when any family member is suffering—emotionally or physically. If this is a situation that applies to your family, family counseling is strongly recommended. The family-systems approach is practiced predominantly by social workers.

Good parenting requires both *time* and *consistency* in order to impart the values that you would like to instill in your children. Putting in time as a parent includes being with them on a regular basis and making an effort to get to know them better. What are their talents? What do they enjoy doing? What are they thinking about and how do they feel? Learning the answers to such questions can pay big dividends for both you and your children. In fostering their growth as individuals, it is essential to give them greater power and responsibility by allowing them to make some of their own decisions. By allowing your child to participate to a greater extent in decision-making, you will also instill confidence and trust, both in themselves and in you.

Other ways to spend time as a family are to worship together each week at church or synagogue and to designate a regularly scheduled time during the weekend for a fun activity. Take turns allowing each member to choose the activity for the day. It can be a powerful confidence-builder. My adult daughters still talk about the family bike rides when, shortly after learning to ride two-wheelers, they would lead the four of us on a route of their choosing. The value of such play cannot be overemphasized. Having fun together as a family strengthens the bonds of love between each family member and defuses whatever stress or other problems may have built up during the week. Even if you cannot be with your child daily (due to being away on business or divorce, for instance), spending consistent time with them on a regular basis will help them experience the world and live their lives with the security, confidence, and caring that comes from their knowing that you love them. Despite all of its inherent struggles and perils, parenting is first and foremost an incredible gift. Appreciating that gift by regularly interacting with your children is one of the most potent means for creating community and fostering both spiritual and social healing that you will ever have.

SUPPORT GROUPS

As a society we are plagued by social ills, most notably divorce rates that top 50 percent, a general sentiment of feeling overworked, dual-career marriages, increasing single-parent families, and a generation of children more adrift and alone than any that has preceded them. At the same time, a movement is afoot in America toward a greater sense of community in response to the silent epidemic of isolation and loneliness that affects so many of us. As a result there has been a significant increase in support groups for those sharing common values, experiences, and goals. Support groups for couples, divorced people, single parents, men, women, people with an illness in common (especially cancer), and people recovering from alcohol and drug addiction—and other addictions—are gathering all over the country. Many of them are affiliated with a church or synagogue, with the added purpose of enhancing spiritual growth. They meet regularly—weekly, every other week, or every month—and the participants by and large report that they benefit from the social connection they find there. If you would like to participate in such a group, most likely you can find them in your local Yellow Pages, or you can contact organizations such as your local United Way, Catholic Charities, AA group, and so on. Many communities also have support groups devoted to specific diseases, and can also be found on the Internet.

Recent scientific research also verifies that support groups can play an important role in helping people with chronic disease. David Spiegel, M.D., conducted a study at Stanford University School of Medicine on women with metastatic breast cancer. All of the women received chemotherapy or radiation therapy. One-half of them were in a support group that met weekly for one year. These women lived twice as long as those who were not in a support group, and three were still alive ten years later.

8. Forgiveness

To err is human; to forgive, divine. —ALEXANDER POPE

I have saved the most challenging but probably the most powerful of the *essential 8* for last. The practice of forgiveness can generate profound health benefits. Intimate relationships and unconditional love cannot exist without forgiveness. How often do you blame yourself for your past actions and mistakes? How often do you blame others for your own problems, stress, or slights (both real and imagined) against you? Forgiveness cancels the demands that you or others *should* have done things differently. Hanging on to these demands changes nothing but keeps us under stress. Refusing to forgive yourself or others keeps you locked into limiting patterns from your past, unable to mobilize the creative power in your life here and now.

The next time you find yourself blaming others, physically point your index finger at them or their images and take a look at where the other three fingers of your hand are pointed. Right back at you! Forgiveness, therefore, begins with accepting responsibility for the role you play in shaping your life's experiences. Only after you begin to forgive yourself can you truly forgive others.

A key first step in your journey of forgiveness is the recognition that you are always doing the best you can at any given moment, in accordance with your awareness at the time. This is true of everyone else as well. All of us make mistakes, and all of us ideally learn from them. You may even choose to believe that there are no mistakes, only lessons. In that moment your action or behavior was based upon past experience, environment, and heredity. You can, however, consciously choose to be different in the future. To continue to blame yourself or someone else for something that occurred in the past is energy depleting and keeps you from moving forward with your life.

Forgiving yourself may be your greatest challenge. No doubt there are a number of things in your past that you regret or for which you feel shame. (For me, parenting mistakes have been the most difficult to forgive.) But wouldn't it be healthier to look at what you can learn from your mistake or painful lesson so that it's not repeated; forgive yourself unconditionally for not knowing more or not performing well enough; and be grateful for this opportunity to learn to do better or change your behavior? A tennis player who misses a shot he thinks he should have made will lose his confidence and ultimately his match if he doesn't quickly recognize what he did wrong, forgive himself, and move on to play the next point. Similarly, we lose the ability to focus and do as well as we know we are capable of doing in the present if we do not forgive ourselves and let go of the past.

The more you are able to do this for yourself, the better you will be able to forgive others. *Remember, you are forgiving the actor, not the action.* You are not condoning cruelty, insensitivity, or incompetence; you are forgiving the offending person. By doing so, you are freeing yourself to move out of the past into the healing present. Anger is the problem; forgiveness is the solution.

Bear in mind, however, that the people you decide to forgive may not choose to accept your forgiveness. Although their refusal to do so can be hurtful, their choice should be respected. What matters is that you are taking the step to heal the relationship. The act of forgiveness takes place within your own psyche and the person you are forgiving may therefore be totally unaware of your action. Or you may be forgiving someone who is deceased. Be realistic and don't set your sights too high: Begin with someone who has been critical of you or guilty of another relatively minor offense. Forgiving others does not necessarily mean that your relationship with them will change, but forgiving them will enable you to feel a greater sense of wholeness. Your relationship with the people you forgive may remain the same on the surface, but it doesn't mean that healing hasn't taken place. You will know it when you feel it.

FRIENDSHIP

A 1997 study from Carnegie-Mellon University in Pittsburgh found that people with a greater diversity of relationships were less likely to get colds. Those with six or more social ties (family, friends, coworkers, neighbors, etc.) were four times *less* susceptible to colds than those with one to three types of relationships. Researchers found that it was not the number of people in the social network that was the important factor, but the diversity. To varying degrees, most of these types of relationships can be called *friendships*.

As children and teenagers, most of us had a number of friends with whom we enjoyed sharing the day's adventures. Our friends helped us meet such challenges as each new year at school, sports, puberty, dating, family problems, and the existential concerns through which all of us passed during our journey into adulthood. Between kindergarten and college, sustaining friendships was made easier by the fact that our friends provided us with a sense of belonging, a feeling of "being in this together," and offered us a forum in which to mutually discuss the problems and issues we faced at the time. Because of such friendships, many people regard the times they spent in high school and college as the happiest days of their lives. Once past college, as they entered the workforce, got married, and juggled the responsibilities of their careers and families, a large segment of our society has lost track of their friends from the past and have not replaced them with new friends.

While most adults enjoy the company of neighbors, coworkers, and other acquaintances, by the time we reach our thirties, studies reveal that those of us who still have a best friend in whom we can confide are exceptionally rare. This is particularly true of men who, because of this lack of a confidant, experience feelings of isolation and absence of support, no matter how fulfilled they may otherwise be in their personal lives and careers.

If you find yourself in need of a good friend, realize that it's never too late to rekindle old friendships or to make new ones. All that is required is a willingness to take risks and make the effort. Having a close friend you can talk to from your heart can provide many additional blessings in your life and deepen your connection with Spirit.

SELFLESS ACTS AND ALTRUISM

Remember a time when you stopped to spontaneously help someone, either a friend or a total stranger? Such selfless acts of giving go to the essence of Spirit, which is always with us, supporting our lives while asking for nothing in return. *Sharing* with others your time, help, and special gifts and talents in ways that benefit them provides you with perhaps the most powerful means of engaging and expressing Spirit and enhancing social health. The opportunities for sharing are abundant and may include donating clothes or money to worthy charities, volunteering time at a homeless shelter, soup kitchen, or after-school tutoring program, or simply setting aside our own tasks and concerns to address the needs of our spouses or children. (There is a great deal of truth in the adage "Charity begins at home.") Another form of sharing that is regaining popularity is *tithing*. Dating back to biblical times, tithing is the practice of donating a certain percentage (usually 5 to 10 percent) of one's yearly income to charity. Interestingly, many people who adopt the practice of tithing also find that their incomes actually begin to increase, although that should not be your motivation for doing so. However you choose to perform selfless acts, remember that the truest form of giving is one that does not call attention to the giver. As Jesus instructed in the Gospel of Matthew, "When you give to the needy, do not announce it with trumpets." The purpose of sharing is *to share,* not to acquire praise or honors. Sharing selflessly will deepen your awareness of how abundantly Spirit is giving to you.

The late Hans Selye, a pioneer in modern stress research, thought that by helping people you earn their gratitude and affection, and that the warmth that results protects against stress. Today, Selye's belief is borne out by mounting evidence that selfless acts not only feel good but are healthy. Epidemiologist James House and his colleagues at the University of Michigan's Survey Research Center studied more than 2,700 men in Tecumseh, Michigan, for almost fourteen years to see how social relationships affected mortality rates. Those who did regular volunteer work had death rates two and one half times lower than those who didn't. The highest form of selfishness is selflessness. When we freely choose to help others, we seem to get as much as, or more than, what we give.

The closer our contact with those we help, the greater the benefits seem to be. Most of us need to feel that we matter to someone, a need that volunteer work can fulfill. There is a growing number of people requiring help in our society, including the homeless, the elderly, the hungry, runaways, orphans, and the illiterate, and there are many ways to help them. Choose to do so in the way that most compels you, but recognize that altruism works best when it comes from the heart and is not calculated as a means to receive something in return.

SUMMARY

Your spiritual well-being is ultimately the most important aspect of your ability to care for yourself. It is also the dimension of holistic medicine that is most often neglected in our society. Becoming spiritually healthy is a process of *diminishing fear and increasing love while developing an awareness of soul and Spirit and allowing It to guide you to a deeper connection to other human beings.* This infinite source of compassionate and forgiving transcendent power is the essence of all life on earth and is the spark of life-force energy within each of us. The most direct path to becoming spiritually healthy is learning to love yourself. As you do, you will appreciate greater meaning and purpose of your life, experience gratitude for your many blessings, and become highly attuned to and trusting of your intuition. As you move beyond the confining restraints of your ego, you will become a more loving friend, spouse or committed partner, parent, and member of your community. In short, you will achieve the goal of holistic medicine: *to become whole,* and to experience a quality of life beyond anything you've probably ever imagined. Or at least beyond a score of 325 on the Thriving Self-Test.

REFERENCES

1. Binder W, Brin M, et al., Botulinum toxin (botox) for treatment in migraine headache: an open label assessment. *Headache,* 344, May 1999.
2. Blanchard E, et al., Five year prospective follow-up on the treatment of chronic headache with biofeedback and/or relaxation. *Headache,* 27:580–583, 1987.
3. Diamond S, Montrose M, The value of biofeedback in the treatment of chronic headache: A four-year retrospective study. *Headache,* 24:5–18, January 1984.
4. Faccinetti F, et al., Magnesium prophylaxis of menstrual migraine: Effects on intracellular magnesium. *Headache,* 31:298–304, 1991.
5. Fontes Ribeiro C, L-5-Hydroxytryptophan in the prophylaxis of chronic tension-type headache: A double-blind, randomized, placebo-controlled study. *Headache,* 40:451–456, June 2000.
6. Johnson ES, et al., Efficacy of feverfew as prophylactic treatment of migraine. *British Med J,* 291:569–737 1985.
7. Klapper J, Mathew N, et al., A multicenter, double-blind, placebo-controlled trial of two dosages of botox (Botulinum Toxin, Type A) in the prophylactic treatment of migraine. *Headache,* 361–362, May 1999.

8. Lundeberg T, Acupuncture in headache. *Cephalalgia,* 19: Suppl 25, 65–68, 1999.

9. Mauskop A, Grossmann W, Schmidramsl H, *Petasites hybridus* (butterbur root) extract is effective in the prophylaxis of migraines: Results of a randomized, double-blind trial. *Headache,* 40:6:420, May 2000.

10. McGrady A, et al., Effect of biofeedback-assisted relaxation on migraine headache and changes in cerebral blood flow velocity in the middle cerebral artery. *Headache,* 34:424–428, July/August 1994.

11. Melchart D, Linde, et al., Acupuncture for recurrent headaches: a systematic review of randomized controlled trial. *Cephalalgia,* 19:779–786, November 1999.

12. Murphy J, et al., Randomized double-blind placebo-controlled trial of feverfew in migraine prevention. *Lancet,* ii:189–192, 1988.

13. Peikert A, Prophylactic of migraine with oral magnesium: results from a prospective, multicenter, placebo-controlled and double-blind randomized study. *Cephalalgia,* 16:257–263, 1996.

14. Pfaffenrath V, et al., Magnesium in the prophylaxis of migraine—a double-blind, placebo-controlled study. *Cephalalgia,* 16:436–440, 1996.

15. Ramadan N, et al., Low brain magnesium in migraine. *Headache,* 29:590–593, 1989.

16. Schoenen J, et al., Effectiveness of high dose riboflavin in migraine prophylaxis. A randomized, controlled trial. *Neurology,* 50:466–470, 1998.

17. Schoenen J, et al., High-dose riboflavin as a prophylactic treatment of migraine: results an open pilot study. *Cephalalgia,* 14:328–329, 1994.

18. Wagner W, Nootbarr-Wagner U, Prophylactic treatement of migraine with gamma-linolenic and alpha-linoleic acids. *Cephalalgia,* 17:127–130, April 1997.

19. Walach H, Haeusler W, et al., Classical homeopathic treatment of chronic headaches. *Cephalalgia,* 17:129–125, 1997.

20. Wauquier A, et al., Changes in cerebral blood flow velocity associated with biofeedback-assisted relaxation treatment of migraine headaches are specific for the middle cerebral artery. *Headache,* 35:358–362, June 1995.
21. Weaver K, Magnesium and migraine. *Headache* 30:168, 1990.

GENERAL TEXTS

1. Mauskop A, Brill M, *The Headache Alternative. A Neurologist's Guide to Drug Free Relief,* Dell Publishing, 1997.
2. Milne R, More B, Goldberg B, *An Alternative Medicine Definitive Guide to Headaches,* Future Medicine Publishing, Inc., 1997.
3. Robbins R, *Management of Headache and Headache Medications,* Second Edition, Springer-Verlag New York, Inc., 2000.
4. Saper J, Silberstein S, et al., *Handbook of Headache Management: A Practical Guide to Diagnosis and* Treatment of Head, Neck, and Facial Pain, Second Edition, Lippincott Williams & Wilkins Inc., 1999.

RESOURCE GUIDE

For more information about the Headache Survival Program or to make an appointment with Dr. Nelson, please contact www. ThrivingHealth.com or call 1-888-434-0033.

The following organizations offer additional information about various aspects of the Headache Survival Program, and provide referrals to practitioners of the many therapies that contribute to this holistic approach for treating, preventing, and curing headache.

HOLISTIC MEDICINE

American Board of Holistic Medicine (ABHM)

(425) 741-2996
Fax (425) 787-8040
www.amerboardholisticmed.com

The ABHM is the first organization to certify physicians in holistic medicine (December 2000 was the first certification examination) and to create the standard of care for holistic medical practice. Provides a referral list of board-certified holistic physicians.

American Holistic Medical Association (AHMA)
6728 Old McLean Village Drive
McLean, VA 22101-3906
(703) 556-9728
Fax (703) 556-8729
www.holisticmedicine.org (a physician referral directory is available)

The nation's oldest advocacy group (founded in 1978) devoted to promoting, teaching, and researching holistic medicine. Provides a list of referrals nationwide of holistic physicians (M.D.s and D.O.s) (available on the website).

OSTEOPATHIC MEDICINE

American Academy of Osteopathy
3500 DePauw Blvd., Suite 1080
Indianapolis, IN 46268
(317) 879-1881

Affiliate organization representing D.O.s who provide osteopathic manipulative treatments and/or cranial osteopathy as part of their practice.

CRANIOSACRAL THERAPY

Cranial Academy
8606 Allisonville Road, Suite 130
Indianapolis, IN 46268
(317) 594-0411
Fax (317) 594-0411/Fax (317) 594-9299

Provides information and a referral list of craniosacral therapists.

Upledger Institute
11211 Prosperity Farms Road
Palm Beach Gardens, FL 33410
(407) 622-4706
Fax (407) 622-4771

Offers training, information, and referrals.

ACUPUNCTURE/TRADITIONAL CHINESE MEDICINE

American Association for Oriental Medicine
433 Front Street
Catasauqua, PA 18032
(610) 266-1433
Fax (610) 264-2768

Professional association for non-M.D. acupuncturists. Offers publications and referral directory of members nationwide.

American Academy of Medical Acupuncture
58200 Wilshire Blvd., Suite 500
Los Angeles, CA 90036
(213) 937-5514

Professional association of physician acupuncturists (M.D.s and D.O.s). Provides educational materials, postgraduate courses, and a membership directory of members nationwide.

National Commission for the Certification of Acupuncturists
1424 16th Street NW, Suite 601
Washington, DC 20036
(202) 232-1404

Provides information about acupuncture and offers a test used by various states to determine competency of acupuncture practitioners.

National Acupuncture Detoxification Association
3115 Broadway, Suite 51
New York, NY 10027
(212) 993-3100

Leading organization of its kind. Conducts research on, and provides training in, the use of acupuncture to treat addiction, including alcoholism.

Qigong Institute/East-West Academy of Healing Arts
450 Sutter Street, Suite 916
San Francisco, CA 94108
(415) 788-2227

Provides education, training, and research about qigong in relation to health and healing.

BEHAVIORAL MEDICINE/MIND-BODY MEDICINE

**National Institute for the Clinical Application
of Behavioral Medicine**
P.O. Box 523
Mansfield Center, CT 06250
(860) 456-1153
Fax (860) 423-4512

Provides conferences and information for practitioners.

Association for Humanistic Psychology
45 Franklin Street, Suite 315
San Francisco, CA 94102
(415) 864-8850

Provides publications about humanistic psychology and a list of referrals.

Center for Mind-Body Medicine
5225 Connecticut Avenue NW, Suite 414
Washington, DC 20015
(202) 966-7338

An educational program for health and mental health professionals, and laypeople interested in exploring their own capacities for self-knowledge and self-care. Provides educational and support groups for people with chronic illness, stress-management groups, and training and programs in mind-body health care.

Mind/Body Medical Institute
New Deaconess Hospital
185 Pilgrim Road
Boston, MA 02215
(617) 632-9530

Provides research, training, and conferences related to behavioral medicine, stress reduction, yoga, and meditation.

BODYWORK/MASSAGE THERAPIES

American Massage Therapy Association
820 Davis Street, Suite 100
Evanston, IL 60201
(312) 761-2682

Provides comprehensive information on most areas of bodywork and massage, including an extensive review of the latest scientific research. Also publishes Massage Therapy Journal, *available at most health food stores and many newsstands nationwide.*

Associated Bodywork and Massage Professionals
P.O. Box 489
Evergreen, CO 80439
(303) 674-8478

Provides information and referrals.

ROLFING

International Rolf Institute
302 Pearl Street
Boulder, CO 80306
(303) 449-5903

Provides information, training, and referral directory.

REFLEXOLOGY

International Institute of Reflexology
P.O. Box 12462
St. Petersburg, FL 33733
(813) 343-4811

Provides information, training, and referrals.

CHIROPRACTIC

American Chiropractic Association
1701 Clarendon Blvd.
Arlington, VA 22209
(703) 276-8800

Professional association offering education and research into chiropractic. Also offers publications.

International Chiropractors Association
1110 North Glebe Road, Suite 1000
Arlington, VA 22201
(800) 423-4690
(703) 528-5000

Professional association offering education and research into chiropractic. Also offers publications.

DIET AND NUTRITION

American College for Advancement in Medicine (ACAM)
23121 Verdugo Drive, Suite 204
Laguna Hills, CA 92653
(800) 532-3688

ACAM provides information about the use of nutritional supplements and a referral directory of physicians worldwide who have been trained in nutritional medicine.

American College of Nutrition
722 Robert E. Lee Drive
Wilmington, NC 28480
(919) 452-1222

Information resource for nutrition research.

Center for Science in the Public Interest
1875 Connecticut Avenue NW, Suite 300
Washington, DC 20009
(202) 332-9110/Fax (202) 265-4954

Provides a directory of organic mail-order suppliers, hormone-free beef suppliers, and general information on diet and nutrition.

American Dietetic Association
216 West Jackson Street, Suite 800
Chicago, IL 60606
(312) 899-0040

Provides information and certification.

International Association of Professional Natural Hygienists
Regency Health Resort and Spa
2000 South Ocean Drive
Hallandale, FL 33009
(305) 454-2220

Professional organization of physicians who specialize in therapeutic fasting.

Great Smokies Diagnostic Laboratory
63 Zillicoa Street
Asheville, NC 28801-1074
(800) 522-4762

Offers fully certified advanced assessments using more than 100 diagnostic tests of digestive, immune, endocrine, nutritional, and metabolic function—supported by a comprehensive network of educational and scientific resources.

ENERGY MEDICINE

International Society for the Study of Subtle Energies and Energy Medicine (ISSSEEM)
356 Goldco Circle
Golden, CO 80401
(303) 278-2228/Fax (303) 279-3539

Research organization; provides education and information, as well as publications.

THERAPEUTIC TOUCH

Nurse Healers Professional Associates, Inc.
1211 Locust Street
Philadelphia, PA 19107
(215) 545-8079

Provides information on training, conferences, and referrals of TT practitioners. Also publishes a newsletter.

HEALING TOUCH

Healing Touch International, Inc.
198 Union Blvd., Suite 204
Lakewood, CO 80228
(303) 989-7982/Fax (303) 985-9702/E-mail: ccheal@aol.com

Provides information and referrals.

REIKI

Reiki Alliance
P.O. Box 41
Cataldo, ID 83810
(208) 682-3535

Provides information and referrals.

ENERGY DEVICES

Tools For Exploration
9755 Independence Avenue
Chatsworth, CA 91311
(888) 748-6657

Provides nonmedical energy machines and other devices. Free catalog available by request.

ENVIRONMENTAL MEDICINE

American Academy of Environmental Medicine
7701 E. Kellogg Street, Suite 625
Wichita, KS 67202
(316) 684-5500

Provides referral list of physicians practicing environmental medicine, as well as a newsletter and other information.

Human Ecology Action League (HEAL)
P.O. Box 49126
Atlanta, GA 30359
(404) 248-1898

Provide referrals to support groups that assist people suffering from environmental illness.

Immuno Labs
1620 West Oakland Park Blvd., Suite 300
Fort Lauderdale, FL 33311
(800) 321-9197

A lab specializing in allergy testing. Also provides referrals to environmental physicians worldwide.

HERBAL MEDICINE

American Botanical Council
P.O. Box 201660
Austin, TX 78720
(512) 331-8868

A nonprofit research organization and education council that serves as a clearinghouse of information for professionals and laypeople alike.

Herb Research Foundation
1007 Pearl Street
Boulder, CO 80302
(303) 449-2265

Provides research information and referrals to resources on botanical medicine worldwide. Also publishes HerbalGram.

HOMEOPATHY

International Foundation for Homeopathy
2366 Eastlake Avenue East, Suite 301
Seattle, WA 98102
(206) 324-8230

Provides training in homeopathy and offers referrals.

National Center for Homeopathy
801 North Fairfax Street, Suite 306
Alexandria, VA 22314
(703) 548-7790

Offers training in homeopathy and provides referrals.

NATUROPATHIC MEDICINE

American Association of Naturopathic Physicians
2366 Eastlake Avenue East, Suite 322
Seattle, WA 98102
(206) 323-7610

Provides information, publications, and a referral directory of naturopathic physicians. Also in the forefront in licensing of naturopaths throughout the United States.

The Institute for Naturopathic Medicine
66½ North State Street
Concord, NH 03301
(603) 255-8844

A nonprofit organization promoting research about naturopathy. Offers information to professionals, laypeople, and the general media.

MEDICAL ASTROLOGY

Jonathan Keyes
(503) 231-9146/E-mail: jonkeyes@qwest.net

PRODUCT INDEX

Magnesium Extra (magnesium glycinate)
Super Potency Essential Fatty Acids (omega-3 oils, EPA and DHA)
Healthy Head Support (boswellia, curcumin, and ginger)
Herbal Muscle Relief (valerian, passionflower, magnesium and calcium)
Herbal Muscle Relief PM (valerian, passionflower, magnesium, calcium, kava kava, and hops)
Petadolex (standardized butterbur extract)
Hepataplex (Chinese herbs)

INDEX

Index

Index

ABOUT THE AUTHORS

Robert S. Ivker, D.O.

Dr. Ivker is a holistic family physician and healer. He began practicing family medicine in Denver in 1972, after graduating from the Philadelphia College of Osteopathic Medicine. He completed a family practice residency at Mercy Medical Center in Denver and was certified by the American Board of Family Practice (ABFP) from 1975 to 1988. For the past 14 years his holistic medical practice has focused on the treatment of chronic disease and the creation of optimal health. He is an Assistant Clinical Professor in the Department of Family Medicine and a Clinical Instructor in the Department of Otolaryngology at the University of Colorado School of Medicine. Dr. Ivker is a co-founder and President-elect of the American Board of Holistic Medicine (ABHM) and cocreator of the first board certification examination in holistic medicine in December 2000. He was the President of the American Holistic Medical Association (AHMA) from 1996 to 1999. Along with the four editions of the best-selling *Sinus Survival: The Holistic Medical Treatment for Sinusitis, Allergies, and Colds,* Dr. Ivker is the coauthor of *The Self-Care Guide to Holistic Medicine: Creating Optimal Health* and *Thriving: The Holistic Guide to Optimal Health for Men. Headache Survival* is part of a Survival Guide series that also includes *Arthritis Survival, Backache Survival,* and *Asthma Survival,* all published by Tarcher/

Putnam in 2001 and 2002. He has been married for thirty-three years to Harriet, a psychiatric social worker; they have two daughters—Julie and Carin—and live in Littleton, Colorado.

Todd H. Nelson, N.D., D.Sc.

Dr. Nelson is a naturopathic doctor and director of the Tree of Life Wellness Center, Colorado's busiest naturopathic clinic. His specialty is clinical nutrition and functional medicine. He has been serving the Denver/Boulder community for eighteen years, integrating comprehensive holistic health care through balanced, educational approaches to self-care. Dr. Nelson lectures extensively on a broad range of holistic health topics, both locally and nationally. He also teaches a corporate wellness program, Stress Mastery, to major corporations. He is the cohost of a popular nationally syndicated radio show, Get Healthy!, on KHOW, Colorado's #1 weekly talk show on holistic medicine. Todd lives in Denver with his wife, Dixie, and four daughters.